"This book provides an excellent overview of current psychoanalytic exploration of the various forms of trauma. It emphasizes that when confronted with the traumatic effects of external destructive events, we must never lose sight of the multiple intrapsychic meaning of traumatic experience. Contributors provide us with new knowledge, and with their extensive clinical material they deepen our insights for treatment. The book helps the psychoanalytic clinician bridge the gap between the theoretical framework of trauma and clinical practice."

—**Werner Bohleber**, Training and Supervising Analyst,
German Psychoanalytical Association

"This collection of essays on trauma, broadly and deeply conceived, is a very welcome addition to trauma studies. The types of trauma being written about – to body, to mind, to infant, to social group – suggest how wide we must set our lens if we are to say something genuinely crucial and helpful to those of us who see trauma in the consulting room. Most importantly, this book exposes the wide range of theories and practices in which trauma work is being done. This marks a very significant shift in psychoanalytic theory and practice. Trauma work can be undertaken with care, with precision and with power, across different theoretical traditions. This is a unifying force in psychoanalysis, and I might say, is the deep message of this collection."

—**Adrienne Harris**, New York University

"For all who are interested in learning from different clinical and theoretical perspectives, this book shows a vast array of well-regarded psychoanalysts' experience in dealing with Trauma – '*a wound that alters development, disrupts time, obstructs symbolization*', as stated by M. Murphy, one of the book's editors. It's really a compilation of a comprehensive psychoanalytic approach to trauma nowadays. I felt so enriched by this truly original and important work and would highly recommend it!."

—**Sergio Nick**, Adult, Child and Adolescent Psychoanalyst,
Brazilian Psychoanalytic Society, Rio de Janeiro,
and Vice President of the International
Psychoanalytical Association

Trauma and the Destructive-Transformative Struggle

The impact of trauma can be both destructive and transformative. This important new book presents not only a range of theoretical frameworks through which different trauma can be understood, from the effects of childhood abuse to those of war and catastrophes, but also gives readers insights into how trauma presents itself in the consulting room.

In each chapter the author uses clinical vignettes and detailed case histories to discuss the multiplicity and complexity of the trauma involved, eschewing a simple binary conception of internal vs external forces. A wide range of topics are covered, including: the lasting imprint of early trauma such as neglect or abuse on subsequent development; the somatic solution involved in life-threatening illness; unmetabolized mourning and embodied memory; the vibrating relationship between catastrophic external forces such as intergenerational effects; and the 9/11 terrorist attacks and the lasting effect of war on combatants and their families.

Each chapter is screened through a different theoretical viewpoint, from Freud and Fairburn to Winnicott, Bion and Ogden, while the work of several contemporary theorists is also discussed. Crucially, the final section of the book looks at those issues faced by analysts when working with traumatized patients, highlighting the key idea of dissociation, the dilemma around empathy and the factors that affect the patient's unconscious meaning.

Trauma and the Destructive-Transformative Struggle: Clinical Perspectives illuminates the resilience needed by both patient and analyst. It will be a vital resource for both clinical practitioners specializing in trauma and psychoanalytic researchers in the field of trauma studies.

Terrence McBride is a Training and Supervising Analyst and Faculty Member at the Los Angeles Institute and Society for Psychoanalytic Studies (LAISPS). He is also Past President and former Dean and Director of Training at LAISPS. He is on the Board of the North American Psychoanalytic Confederation (NAPsaC) and is the current President of the Confederation of Independent Psychoanalytic Societies (CIPS). He is in private practice in Los Angeles, California.

Maureen Murphy is a Personal and Supervising Analyst and Faculty Member at the Psychoanalytic Institute of Northern California (PINC). She was the Founding President of PINC and former chair of NAPsaC. She teaches courses on contemporary psychosomatic concepts, particularly the impact of burgeoning biotechnology on core psychoanalytic concepts. She is in private practice in San Francisco.

Trauma and the Destructive-Transformative Struggle

Clinical Perspectives

Edited by
Terrence McBride and Maureen Murphy

Routledge
Taylor & Francis Group
LONDON AND NEW YORK

First published 2020
by Routledge
2 Park Square, Milton Park, Abingdon, Oxon OX14 4RN

and by Routledge
52 Vanderbilt Avenue, New York, NY 10017

Routledge is an imprint of the Taylor & Francis Group, an informa business

British Library Cataloguing in Publication Data
A catalogue record for this book is available from the British Library

Library of Congress Cataloging-in-Publication Data
A catalog record has been requested for this book

ISBN: 978-0-367-33389-8 (hbk)
ISBN: 978-0-367-33390-4 (pbk)
ISBN: 978-0-429-31958-7 (ebk)

Typeset in Times New Roman
by Taylor & Francis Books

In memory of
Ernest S. Lawrence, Ph.D.,
Analyst, Mentor, Colleague, Friend
with enduring gratitude

Contents

Acknowledgments

We wish to express our appreciation to all of the contributors to this book for providing a rich and diverse cross section of examples of trauma. In each chapter, they present vivid and in-depth illustrations of the psychoanalytic process in the treatment of the multiple manifestations of trauma in the clinical situation.

We are grateful to the Book Series Program of the Confederation of Independent Psychoanalytic Societies (CIPS), The Boundaries of Psychoanalysis, and to its editor, Fredric Perlman, for giving us the opportunity to bring this book to fruition. All of the myriad aspects involved in the preparation of this manuscript have been an inspiring and meaningful experience.

We also thank the publishing staff at Routledge, especially Russell George and Elliott Morsia, for their guidance and support in the publication of this book.

We want to acknowledge the contributions of colleagues Linda Sobelman, Andrea Kahn, Alan Spivak, Linda Weitzman, Robin Deutsch and Harvey Peskin for their generative input.

Finally, we wish to thank our loved ones for their emotional support during the long process of making this book a reality. Terrence thanks his wife, Linda Sobelman, for her love and patient understanding; his adult children, Terry, Coleen, Brigitte and Michael; and a special expression of appreciation goes to his sister, Rita McBride, for her constant love and encouragement.

Maureen thanks her husband, Joel Fruchtman, for his unwavering confidence in her and this project, for rescuing her from computer madness and for ever-inspired editing.

Contributors

Terrence McBride, Psy.D., FIPA, BCPsa, co-editor of this volume, is a Training and Supervising Analyst and Faculty Member at the Los Angeles Institute and Society for Psychoanalytic Studies (LAISPS), where he is also Past President and former Dean and Director of Training. He is a former Faculty Member at the Wright Institute Los Angeles, and was a founding member of the Los Angeles Chapter of the American Association for Psychoanalysis in Clinical Social Work. He is on the board of the North American Psychoanalytic Confederation (NAPsaC), and has served on the board and is a two-term Vice President and current President of the Confederation of Independent Psychoanalytic Societies (CIPS). His most recent publication is a chapter in the book, *Battling the Life and Death Forces of Sadomasochism: Clinical Perspectives* (Karnac, 2013). He is in private practice in Los Angeles, California.

Maureen Murphy, Ph.D., BCPsa, co-editor of this volume, is a Personal and Supervising Analyst and Faculty Member at the Psychoanalytic Institute of Northern California (PINC), where she was the founding President and is the current co-chair of its Distance Learning Program. She is the former chair of NAPsaC, a two-term North American representative to the IPA board and a board member of CIPS. She teaches courses on contemporary psychosomatic concepts, particularly the impact of burgeoning biotechnology on core psychoanalytic concepts. She is in private practice in San Francisco.

Maxine K. Anderson, M.D., FIPA, is a founding member of the Northwestern Psychoanalytic Society and Institute (NPSI) in Seattle, Washington, where she is a Training and Supervising Analyst. She is also a Training and Supervising Analyst with the Seattle Psychoanalytic Society and Institute and the Canadian Psychoanalytic Society, and a Fellow of the British Psychoanalytic Society. She has written widely on various topics. Her most recent book is *From Tribal Division to Welcoming Inclusion: Psychoanalytic Perspectives* (Routledge, 2019), which deals with the need to maintain self-respecting whole-mindedness in order to deal responsibly with the current tendencies toward polarization and hatred of otherness.

Susan S. Berger, Psy.D., FIPA, is an Adult Psychoanalyst and Psychotherapist in New York City, working as well with children and adolescents and their families. A graduate and Training and Surpervising Analyst of the Institute of Psychoanalytic Training and Research (IPTAR) in Adult Psychoanalysis, she is a member of the institute's board of directors. She is a former Co-Director and is currently on the Faculty and Executive Committee of its Child and Adolescent Psychotherapy (CAP) training program. She is on the steering committee of the Gould Center for Psychoanalytic Organizational Study and Consultation, and completed IPTAR's Socio-Analytic Program in Organizational Consultation and Executive Coaching. Previous publications include 'Whose Trauma is it Anyway? Furthering our Understanding of its Intergenerational Transmission' (*JICAP*) and the co-authored 'On Becoming a Supervisee: Preparing for Learning in a Supervisory Relationship' (*Psychotherapy*). In addition to her interest in intergenerational transmission of trauma and psychoanalytic learning, she has a particular interest, within the realm of child and adolescent psychotherapy, in working with parents.

Fred Busch, Ph.D., FIPA, is a Training and Supervising Analyst at the Boston Psychoanalytic Society and Institute. He has published over 90 articles in the psychoanalytic literature, and three books, primarily on the method and theory of treatment. His work has been translated into eight languages, and he has been invited to present over 160 papers and clinical workshops nationally and internationally. His third book, *Creating a Psychoanalytic Mind: A Method and Theory of Psychoanalysis*, was a finalist for the Gradiva Awards. He has been the editor of *JAPA Books*, and has been on numerous editorial boards.

Michael J. Diamond, Ph.D., FIPA, BCPsa, is a Training and Supervising Analyst and Faculty Member at LAISPS. His major publications are on psychoanalytic technique, fathering, masculinity and gender, as well as trauma and dissociation. His books include the recent CIPS series text, *The Second Century of Psychoanalysis: Evolving Perspectives on Therapeutic Action*, and *My Father Before Me: How Fathers and Sons Influence Each Other Throughout Their Lives.* He has a private practice in Los Angeles, California.

Pamela Dirham, Ph.D., FIPA, BCPsa, is a Clinical Psychologist and Psychoanalyst living in Los Angeles. She is a Training and Supervising Analyst at LAISPS, where she is currently Dean and Director of Training. Her clinical interests include primitive mental states, the effects of trauma in personality development and psyche-soma integration. She is in private practice in Los Angeles, California.

Judy K. Eekhoff, Ph.D., FIPA, BCPsa, is a Licensed Child Psychologist and a Training and Supervising Analyst at NPSI. She is on the editorial board of the *American Journal of Psychoanalysis.* Her writing interests include somatic manifestations of preverbal experience in transference and countertransference. Her most recent book is entitled *Trauma and Primitive Mental States: An Object Relations Perspective* (Routledge, 2019). She has a private practice in Seattle, where she also teaches, writes and consults.

Helen K. Gediman, Ph.D., ABPP, FIPA, BCPsa, is a Clinical Professor of Psychology and Consultant at the New York University Postdoctoral Program in Psychotherapy and Psychoanalysis, and Faculty and Training and Supervising Analyst at the Contemporary Freudian Society. She has also spent 17 years on the board of Section 1, Psychoanalyst-Psychologist Practitioners of the American Psychological Association. She has published and presented over 65 papers and 5 books, including *Building Bridges: The Selected Psychoanalytic Papers of Helen K. Gediman* (IPBooks, 2018) and *Stalker, Hacker, Voyeur, Spy* in the recent CIPS series (Routledge, 2017). She is in full-time private practice in New York City.

Thomas P. Helscher, Ph.D., FIPA, is a Training and Supervising Analyst, Faculty Member and Past President at LAISPS. He is also Past Chair of the Clinical Committee of the Soldiers Project. He teaches in the University of California Veterans' Writing Workshop, and is on the UC Interdisciplinary Psychoanalytic Consortium and the Faculty of the Wright Institute Los Angeles. He is in private practice in Santa Monica, California.

W. Preston Lear, Psy.D., L.C.S.W., is a Senior Candidate at LAISPS. He is a co-founder of Community West, an intensive outpatient treatment program for youth and young adults, located in West Los Angeles. He is in private practice in Los Angeles, California.

Maxine Nelson, L.I.C.S.W., FIPA, is a graduate and current President of NPSI, where she has served in a number of leadership positions, as well as on the Faculty. She is on the board of CIPS and NAPsaC. She has a longstanding interest in the intersection of visual art, including film and psychoanalysis, and has written and presented widely on this topic. She maintains a private practice in Bellevue, Washington, where she provides psychoanalysis and psychoanalytic psychotherapy to adults, as well as clinical consultation.

Lori O'Brien, Ph.D., FIPA, BCPsa, is a Training and Supervising Analyst and Faculty Member at LAISPS, where she is also Past President. She is a former board member of the Wright Institute Los Angeles. She is in private practice in Los Angeles, California.

Robert L. Pyles, M.D., has twice served as President of the American Psychoanalytic Association, President of the Massachusetts Psychiatric Society, two terms on the board of the International Psychoanalytical Association, and is a Training and Supervising Analyst at the Psychoanalytic Society and Institute of New England. He has applied psychoanalytic principles to a variety of other fields, such as serving as an expert legal witness and being a consultant to Major League Baseball.

Marilyn Rifkin, L.C.S.W., FIPA, BCpsa, is a Training and Supervising Analyst and Faculty Member at IPTAR. She is also on the Faculty and supervises at the Metropolitan Institute for Training and Psychoanalytic Psychotherapy (MITPP), and was visiting Faculty at the Westchester Center for the Study of Psychoanalysis and Psychotherapy (WCSPP), New York. She has written and presented on the subjects of transference–countertransference enactment, psychosomatics and trauma. Her most recent publication is a chapter in the book *From Soma to Symbol: Psychosomatic Conditions and Transformative Experience* (Karnac, 2016). She maintains a private practice in New York City and Westchester.

Alan P. Spivak, Ph.D., FIPA, BCPsa, is a Training and Supervising Analyst and Faculty Member at LAISPS, and a Faculty Member at the Wright Institute Los Angeles. He is also a Past President of the Los Angeles Society for Psychoanalytic Psychology. He has published and presented psychoanalytic papers, and lectures nationally and internationally on a range of topics, including psychoanalytic interpretation, the curative aspects of psychoanalysis, child abuse trauma and "stealth" intimacy. At the University of California, Los Angeles (UCLA) he has pioneered psychoanalytic extension courses that outreach to general audiences. He is a two-time recipient of the Sanville Award for creative writing in psychoanalysis.

Introduction

Maureen Murphy

About 25 years ago, a man appeared for his first session carrying a volume of Seamus Heaney. As he began to speak about the reasons that brought him to my office, he opened to a bookmarked page and read a now famous stanza from Heaney's *The Cure at Troy* about the pain we inflict on one another and the hardness that befalls us. He continued: "I know that getting hard could be my fate and I want something different."

Without knowing it, my patient provided as good a definition as any of trauma—a wound that alters development, disrupts time, obstructs symbolization. Trauma replaces perception with a clanging sensation—an experience that "endangers life without the capacity to structure a defense" (Tarantelli, 2003, p. 920).

Trauma, cumulative or acute, leaves little of the major supportive psychic structures—bodily integrity, attachment and agency—untouched.

This book addresses the destructive and transformative potential of trauma based on extensive clinical material that emerged from the jointly sponsored conference by the Confederation of Independent Psychoanalytic Societies (CIPS) and the North American Psychoanalytic Confederation (NAPsaC). The conference, entitled "Trauma, Destruction and Transformative Potential", was held in 2014 during the weekend of the opening of the 9/11 Memorial Museum in New York City.

While trauma is the pentimento upon which most psychoanalytic concepts rest, there has been little agreement about the definition and legitimate use of the word. This led Anna Freud (1967) to ask:

> Do I mean that the event was upsetting, that it was significant for altering the course of future development, that it was pathogenic? Or do I mean trauma in its strictest sense: shattering, devastating, causing internal disruption by putting ego functioning and ego mediation out of action? (pp. 237–238)

Until recently we have been limited by the idea that the primary task of psychoanalysis is, as Arlow (1985) puts it, "skewed in the direction of facilitating the emergence into consciousness of persistent unconscious conflict that originated during childhood" (p. 525). This idea, widely held, privileged the lifting of repression, a solidly symbolic defense, and perpetuated the idea that good enough childhood development should see an individual through whatever else life delivers. This theoretical skew not only isolated trauma theory; it also excluded the impact of social, cultural and political experiences on psychic development.

More recently, psychoanalysis has moved beyond its reliance on the rational—the capacity of the individual to manage their drives in the service of personal satisfaction—to include those realties (developmental, somatic and social political events) that cannot be altered by agency or intentionality. This collection of papers moves beyond the binary internal/external in favor of a dialectic of the material and the dynamic. Trauma is then understood as any situation in which the "raw data of existential experience is not transformed into psychic experience—circumstances that outstrip and disrupt the psyche's capacity for representation and mentalization" (Levine, 2014, p. 219). Poetically expressed by Tarantelli: "A traumatic event in an experiential sense is a paradox—an experience that cannot be experienced" (p. 918).

In this volume, the contributors locate their clinical work in a theoretical framework providing an opportunity for readers to critically examine an array of viewpoints. Among others, Freud, Bion, Fairbairn, Ogden and Winnicott are represented.

In the chapters that follow, all of the patients struggle to manage attachment behaviors, to learn from experience and to balance autonomic arousal with imaginative reconstruction. The fear of being overwhelmed by emotional arousal leads to a troubling dyad of numbness on the one hand and relentless memory persecution on the other. For some, as in early trauma, manifestations are ghost-like, only recognizable by a trail of self-defeating repetitions that keep their lives mired in inner chaos. Others knew that something had happened—illness, violence, rape—yet felt helpless to regain the buoyant optimism of their former lost self. For many the struggle to maintain coherence required distorting time—forbidding links with the past in the present and clouding the future. The future is no longer a given—something to be hoped for.

Particularly important contributions to this volume are a series of papers on social, political catastrophes. As mentioned earlier, the conference from which this volume emerged was held on the eve of the opening of the 9/11 Memorial Museum. Part of the experience of the conference was visiting the site of a major terrorist attack literally on New York City and emotionally on a sense of basic security for the rest of the USA. While the plaza was open to the public that day, only the families of those lost in the attack and first responders were permitted inside.

From the outside, I could see families and first responders as the elevator ascended into the museum—an accidental community brought together not by love but by an act of hatred. The memorial is moving, as befits the enormous loss of human life that it represents. Yet as I stood there, I couldn't be consoled by its beauty—only overwhelmed by trying to find some sense of a good object to hold onto. As I walked back to the meeting, only two blocks away, I got completely lost. I had my cell phone but couldn't remember the name of the hotel. I floated along the street in some sense of trance and panic—the kind of dissociation so well known to characterize trauma. Finally, I found my way back to colleagues that I could talk to about the experience, saving me from one of trauma's great injuries—being helpless and resourceless.

And what about the analyst? The traumatized person or circumstance acts on the analyst in a real way. Each contribution to this volume highlights the dyadic nature of trauma—that the fate of the speaker is inextricably linked to that of the listener/witness. Like all witnesses, analysts must find the resilience to bear hearing terrible stories, unthinkable events, versions of man's inhumanity to man. The analysts describe what Ghislaine Boulanger (2005) calls the inevitable "enactive witnessing"—the task of remaining grounded enough to enter into a therapeutic reverie that permits fantasy, thinking and interpreting when even thinking seems impossible.

At these time, the therapist faces feelings of loss by relentless concretism in place of a rich symbolic collaboration and, most confusingly, by getting lost in an explosion of projections. Now the therapist has to withstand what Feigleson (1993) characterizes as the uncanny in treatment. In his paper 'The Uncanny', Freud (1919) talks about two experiences that are relevant here: the double and the return of the repressed. In these clinical situations, the analyst encounters a category of experience in which the familiar and unfamiliar are eerily entwined. In this mix, the sense of what has happened to the patient has happened or could happen to me. The boundary between the analyst and the patient starts to blur—the patient and therapist become doubles of one another. What gives the uncanny its edginess is the impression that something secretly familiar but usually held in place by repression has returned unbidden and unmetabolized. It is this reunion with our own primitiveness that provokes anxiety in the analyst and the wish to turn away. With the return of the repressed, the horror of the patient acts on the analyst in an immediate way, undoing long-established structures. A childhood ago, the analyst had assembled a reliable body schema from dislocated body parts, images of torn skin, the sensation of falling into pieces and wanting it to stay put, not splinter and fray when least expected.

The transformative potential of treatment rests on the analyst's ability to keep relationships alive for the patient as a counter-traumatic recourse to the good object. The analyst holds in trust a sense of the future even in the face of experiences that represent the negation of psychic life. Restoration of personal authorship (Reisner, 2003), giving voice to a story muted by trauma, is the quest chronicled throughout this volume.

Chapters

Trauma isn't a monolithic phenomenon. It may be the accretion of years of blighted developmental attunement or an unexpected moral or somatic assault. Sometimes the toll is exacted as the repetition of disappointing choices. The body, personal and societal, is a likely site in which to see trauma's intrusion.

The chapters that follow are unique in that they are rich in detailed clinical material. They chronicle the destructive-transformative struggle between patient and analyst, illuminating the resilience needed to transform destruction into potential. Possibly: They chronicle the resilience needed by patient and analyst to transform destruction into potential. The chapters are divided into four sections.

Part I: the legacy of early trauma

This section takes up the lasting imprint of early trauma on subsequent development. Beginning with a wide lens on psychoanalytic perspectives on development, Terrence McBride's chapter, "From the Black Hole to the Last Frontier: The Trauma of Childhood Abuse and the Oedipal Stage of Development", provides the foundation for subsequent chapters on childhood trauma. McBride vividly describes a clinical situation in which the reality of abuse was dissociated, resulting in the obscuring of oedipal dynamics. It was only in the transference that the patient's oedipal development could be reconstructed.

Pamela Dirham and Lori O'Brien describe different manifestations of early maternal neglect. In Dirham's chapter—"The Trauma of Otherness and the Struggle for Connection: Schizoid and Sadomasochistic Defenses against Contact with the Other"—she lets us know that for her patient, Jack, this struggle all but foreclosed the possibility of relational mutuality and professional achievement.

Lori O'Brien's "Stubborn Love" movingly describes the desperate attempts of the infant to secure connection in the face of maternal incompetence. O'Brien's patients repetitively seek romantic connections similar to those of their inadequate caretakers in an effort to provide a more positive outcome.

Judy K. Eekhoff addresses the task the analyst faces when she attempts to enter the world of patients who early on "lost innocence and potential". Often relying only on instinct and intuition, analysts who work with these patients "must answer the … call from the lost mother and become the mother who calls them forth from the silent depths of themselves".

Part II: embodied assaults

Joyce McDougall (1974) proposes that each of us searches for a solution to psychic pain—one of which is the somatic solution. In Part II, the contributors portray the body's somatic solution in all its material and enigmatic manifestations.

Maureen Murphy provides examples of sudden onset trauma occasioned by life-threatening diagnoses. Drawing on the treatment of patients with cancer and cardiac transplantation, she describes the subjective experience of patient and analyst as they shuttle between states of meaning and oblivion. She delineates the contribution that psychoanalysis can make to situations in which actual trauma fundamentally disrupts lives.

W. Preston Lear, in "The Icarus Complex and the Trauma of Falling Forever", uses the canvas of extreme sports to illustrate the dichotomy between an "adaptive, creative" use of the body and an omnipotent, Icarus-like, response to early trauma. Lear proposes that, for some, participation in activities such as BASE jumping and rock climbing may provide a defense against deficient maternal holding. The intentional fall becomes an antidote to being dropped. The treatment situation is saturated with the same manic, self-destructive features. The analyst is inevitably drawn into sadomasochistic enactments that require him to balance his own analytic ambitions lest they both fall together.

In "Psychic Deadness and the Vicissitudes of Unmetabolized Mourning" Maxine Nelson's patient, Sam, presents a different solution for dealing with psychic deadness. When there is a breakdown in a mother's alpha function, coupled with cumulative trauma from paternal abuse and the death of a sibling, the infant must evacuate his unmetabolized emotional experiences. For Sam, his body was the recipient of his rage and grief. Nelson describes the empathic task of the analyst who travels with a patient who relies on nihilism as a form of psychic balance.

Marilyn Rifkin's chapter, "Trauma and Embodied Memory", chronicles the traumatic impact of the failure of maternal child differentiation in which the child existed not as an independent subject but as an extension of her mother. Leveraging Marianne Leuzinger-Bohleber's concept of embodied memory, Rifkin proposes the decoding of bodily experience as a vehicle for understanding early trauma. The patient, Ms. D, had suffered numerous intrusive urological exams secondary to enuresis. Throughout the chapter, the transference–countertransference dynamics are detailed, specifically those that veer toward individuation.

Part III: political catastrophes

Part III explores those circumstances in which the victims of trauma are not only individuals but also countries and, indeed, civilization. These chapters illustrate the vibrating relationship between external forces and intrapsychic life.

In "Trauma and the Fate of Nations" Robert L. Pyles names the psychic consequences engendered by terrorism: "a fear that we can no longer rely on what we thought was real". This is nothing less than an attack on what Erikson describes as the most basic development task, navigating basic trust–nontrust. To answer the question "Why do they hate us so much?" requires that we again confront and bear our own primitive impulses that we had previously quieted by various defensive strategies.

Susan S. Berger's chapter, "Learning to Live with Ghosts: Linking Trauma to an Intergenerational Collective Past", employs several clinical vignettes that advocate for the importance of analytic attention to external reality—historical and present—if we are to understand the intrapsychic life of our patients. She reminds us, echoing Pyles in this volume, that the clinical sensitivity to the destructiveness of one group of people to another inevitably leads to a fear of our own aggression and requires us to find ways to bridge the external and the intrapsychic.

Helen K. Gediman's "Trauma, Destruction and PTSD: Vignettes of Resiliency and Transformative Potential" expands the definition to include the idea that massive trauma overwhelms the capacity to symbolize the relationship between the contemporary situation and past early trauma. Gediman provides three vignettes from the 9/11 terrorist attack that illustrate the vicissitudes encountered when past and present emerge in treatment. Citing Alan Bass, she concludes that what distinguishes a positive or negative therapeutic outcome hinges on the degree to which an inescapable external experience of destruction replicates the person's worst internal arousal—the closer the replication, the more ominous the therapeutic outcome.

The fourth chapter in this section turns to the lasting impact of war on combatants and their families. Thomas P. Helscher's "Moral Injury, the Moral Defense and the Collapse of Emotional Containment: An Intersubjective Alternative to PTSD in the Treatment of Wartime Trauma" moves beyond PTSD to the concept of moral injury. Described as a "sickness of the heart" (Levinson, 2012), moral injury stems from taking part in or witnessing something of consequence that you find wrong, which violates your deeply held beliefs about yourself and the world. Moral injury involves the collapse of the good object—the self and valued institutions—coupled with identification with a bad object. Helscher movingly describes the treatment of a recent veteran struggling to regain the potential for a good object. Borrowing from Coleridge's *Rime of the Ancient Mariner*, the task of the analyst and patient becomes the transformation of raw pain into a dynamic narrative.

Part IV: technical issues/analytic resilience

Historically, approaches to the treatment of trauma have been rife with binary disputes circling around the impact of the traumatic event versus the reactivation of preexisting conflicts and fantasies. More recently, there has been an effort to acknowledge the actuality of the trauma while incorporating interpretation of intrapsychic fantasies and conflicts that influence the experience of the event without pathologizing the traumatized subject. In this section four chapters are devoted to specific technical considerations that attempt to bridge the bifurcation of traumatic experience.

Fred Busch, in "The Clinical Significance and Problems of a Traumaticentric View", argues for a technical stance that "addresses the fantasies conflicts and defenses that inevitably develop in the face of trauma" rather than an exclusively empathic approach. Following Marilia Aisentein, Busch makes the point that inclusion of a patient's psychic development in understanding trauma has the potential to "aid patients in becoming their own agent". Busch offers two extensive examples in which earlier issues of separation colored adult responses to trauma as played out in the transference–countertransference relationship.

Maxine K. Anderson, in "Sources of Internal Psychic Trauma", poetically renders the cost of being drawn into an empathic cocoon for both patient and analyst. At first, Anderson complies with frame-bending requests, only to find herself cast as a "mad old woman" in her patient's dream. The lure of empathy to avoid retraumatization may collapse the space for differentiation. Anderson uses the word "sturdy" to describe the necessary position of the analyst if she is to help her patient regain and retain the capacity to think and to feel human. Anderson advocates for the maintenance of a space that permits thought rather than mutual immobilization.

Dissociation, a central hallmark of all traumatic states, is taken up by Michael J. Diamond in "Treating the Traumatized Mind: Dissociation and Psychoanalytic Technique". He illustrates the way that dissociated memories—the "raw data" of a traumatic experience—allude to symbolization while often hiding out in the body. Diamond uses the example of his exchange with a patient in which he names a dissociated state to show how both he and the patient were then able to think. Diamond concludes: "The analyst's witnessing, experiencing, and suffering—as well as his articulation of the dissociated experience in analytic space—enable the *now-ness* of unconscious, actual (traumatized) time to become partially transferred into psychic representation."

In the concluding chapter, "The Central Role of Unconscious Fantasy in the Analysis of Child Abuse Trauma", Alan P. Spivak provides a case from two time frames in an analysis to illustrate the patient's use of idealized erotic fantasies in the transference to keep at bay fragmented memories of paternal sexual abuse. Spivak describes how the interpretation of erotized longings and collusion with her sexual abuse served to ward off more primitive disturbances in the mother–daughter attachment. Spivak argues that:

> [T]he unconscious meaning which the child gives to its precocious sexual experience, that is, her construal of what is happening to her at the time of the abuse … [is] in turn, co-determined by her character structure, phase of development, family dynamics and internal object world—that is, by factors predating the abuse.

References

Arlow, J. (1985). The concept of psychic reality and related problems. *Journal of the American Psychoanalytical Association*, 33: 521–535.

Boulanger, G. (2005). From voyeur to witness: Recapturing symbolic function after massive psychic trauma. *Psychoanalytic Psychology*, 22(1): 21–31.

Feigleson, C. (1993). Personality death, object loss and the uncanny. *International Journal of Psychoanalysis*, 74: 331–345.

Freud, A. (1967). Comments on psychic trauma. *The Writings of Anna Freud. Volume 5*. New York: International Universities Press, 221–241.

Freud, S. (1919). The uncanny. *The Standard Edition of the Complete Works of Sigmund Freud. Volume XVII: An Infantile Neurosis and Other Works* [hereafter *Standard Edition*]. London: Hogarth Press, 217–256.

Levine, H. (2014). Psychoanalysis and trauma. *Psychoanalytic Inquiry*, 34(3): 214–224.

Levinson, N. (2012) Mad, bad, sad: What's really happened to America's soldiers? *The Nation Institute online* (June 28, 2012).

McDougall, J. (1974). The psychosoma and the psychoanalytic process. *International Review of Psychoanalysis*, 1: 437–459.

Reisner, S. (2003). Psychic trauma and the seduction of the painful past. *Studies in Gender and Sexuality*, 4: 263–286.

Tarantelli, C. (2003). Life with death: Towards a metapsychology of catastrophic psychic trauma. *International Journal of Psychoanalysis*, 84(4): 915–928.

Part I

The legacy of early trauma

Chapter 1

From the black hole to the last frontier

The trauma of childhood abuse and the oedipal stage of development

Terrence McBride

> [T]he boundary of the black hole is like the edge of a shadow—the shadow of impending doom...[it] acts as rather like a one-way membrane around the black hole: objects...can fall through...into the black hole, but nothing can ever get out...One could say...what the poet Dante said of the entrance to Hell: "All hope abandon ye who enter here." Anything or anyone who falls through the [boundary] will soon reach the region of infinite density and the end of time.
>
> Stephen Hawking (1988, pp. 98–99)

Introduction

The purpose of this chapter is to explore the relationship between the trauma of early childhood parental abuse and the dynamics of the oedipal phase of development, elaborating on the reciprocal effects of each on the other. It is based on the case study of a long-term analytic patient, Mr. B, who was verbally and emotionally abused by his father from about the age of two to the age of ten, and inappropriately exposed to incest-inducing fantasies by his mother during latency, which is interpreted as a form of sexual abuse. The interplay between the intrapsychic structural damage of the trauma of both instances of abuse and preexisting and subsequent oedipal conflicts that were in play at the time is the subject of discussion.

Developmental trauma

The concept of developmental trauma disorder has been conceived outside of psychoanalysis in the fields of psychiatry and neurobiology by Van der Kolk (2005) and colleagues as an argument for a rational diagnosis for children with complex trauma histories. Since the majority of traumatized children do not meet the criteria for the DSM-IV diagnosis of post-traumatic stress disorder (PTSD) for adult-onset trauma, it was proposed as an alternative. It is based on the term "complex trauma", which is described as multiple, chronic and prolonged exposure to developmentally adverse traumatic events, most often of an interpersonal nature, with early-life onset. Van der Kolk's comprehensive list of the deleterious effects of childhood trauma on development is consistent with psychoanalytic views of psychopathological consequences from childhood trauma (Fonagy & Target, 2003). Included are disruptions of affect regulation, disturbed attachment patterns, self-hatred and self-blame, aggressive behaviors against self and others, altered schemas of the world, loss of autonomous strivings, chronic feelings of ineffectiveness and failure to achieve developmental competencies (p. 406). It is also noted that, although major, trauma is not the sole factor in developmental disturbance, but is included in a more complex interaction with adequate care and nurturing, as well as biology and genetic constitutional endowment (Malberg & Mayes, 2015). A psychoanalytic view adds the critical element that preexisting unconscious fantasies and intrapsychic conflicts also play a central role in the impact of the trauma and subsequent effects that it may have (Busch, 2005; Sugerman, 2018; Spivak, this volume).

Psychoanalytic perspectives on development

According to Tyson and Tyson (1990), the developmental perspective in psychoanalysis has been present from the beginning. It "has had its own evolution, which parallels the history of psychoanalysis" (p. 2). Anna Freud (1965) stressed the value of looking at personality functioning through a developmental psychoanalytic lens in order to organize diverse aspects of complex clinical phenomena and to permit their full meaning to emerge (p. 328). In spite of those who dispute the importance of a patient's developmental history, most psychodynamic theorists think that understanding development is intrinsic to treatment (Gilmore & Meersand, 2014, p. 4).

Pioneers of early theories of development provide the relevance on which contemporary views of infant and childhood developmental trauma and its detrimental effects are based. These effects can lead to lifelong psychopathology of varying degrees. All authors stress the interactions and interdependencies between maturational and environmental factors. Anna Freud (1965, 1967) conceived of eight lines of development from infancy to adolescence which can be disrupted or impeded by trauma from internal or external forces. Nagera (1966) emphasized the concept of "developmental interference", which involves gross external (environmental) interferences that can disturb the typical unfolding of development before the child's ego capacity is able to cope with them. Erikson's (1950) epigenetic phase-specific developmental tasks emphasize both the challenge and the hazard involved in each developmental stage, beginning with the first stage—the establishment of a sense of basic trust. Although the phases overlap, if the tasks of one phase are insufficiently mastered due to some disturbance, the course and outcome of subsequent stages of development can be affected that persist into adulthood and throughout the life cycle. Mahler et al. (1975) provided a model of the separation–individuation phase of development, ranging from infancy to toddlerhood, requiring the mastery of certain developmental tasks during each of four subphases. Toddlers are especially vulnerable to psychic trauma and overwhelming distress during the rapprochement subphase which can undermine the outcome of the separation–individuation process.

Finally, Bowlby (1969) conceived of a theory of attachment based on the infant's predisposition to attachment. His theory provides a link between earlier models of development and contemporary views of the relationship between trauma and development, especially from the object relations perspective. His critical contribution was the infant's need for unbroken early attachment to the mother (Fonagy & Target, 2003, p. 232) and the trauma of separation if the attachment is disrupted (Bowlby, 1960). Ainsworth et al. (1978) extended Bowlby's model by describing patterns of attachment from secure to insecure attachment. This affects the quality of information processing about the external environment, affect regulation and the capacity for bonding and attachment throughout life, depending on the early provisions for the child's needs.

In the modern view of development, there is disagreement about the linear structure, standard progression and distinct pathways of the classical developmental phases cited above, especially in regard to the oedipal phase because of its transformative function. It is based on the nonlinear dynamics systems model of development (Galatzer-Levy, 1995; Gilmore, 2008). This model views development as a nonlinear, hierarchically ordered perspective on mental organizations that occur in a relatively reliable way across individuals and cultures. "Each phasic shift is the product of multiple interacting systems, none of which can fully realize the given state independently" (Gilmore & Meersand, 2014, p. 2).

Trauma and development

A developmental view has also been present since the beginning of psychoanalysis in regard to trauma. According to Bohleber (2007), "Psychoanalysis began as a theory of trauma" (p. 329). While Freud never developed an organized theory of trauma, it remained a prominent idea in his mind throughout his career. His early theory of the origin of psychoneurosis was based on childhood seduction and childhood sexual trauma (Freud, 1896). He began with the view that the major emotional experience of the trauma of sexual abuse had to be repressed because of its unacceptability to the conscious mind. As a result, the effects induced by the forgotten event continued to press for discharge which caused symptoms. He later revised this view to define trauma as a situation that occurs when the quantity of excitation overwhelms the ego and breaks through the stimulus barrier (Freud, 1920). He developed this idea further in his revised theory of affects, where he defined trauma as the arousal of anxiety of such intensity that the ego's organizing, synthesizing and defensive functions become overwhelmed and render the person helpless (Freud, 1926).

Psychoanalysts have long recognized that childhood traumatic experience can disrupt and impede the child's progression in all periods of development. It can have a profound impact on the capacity to integrate sensory, emotional, cognitive, behavioral and relational information into a cohesive whole. The magnitude of influence that trauma can have on later development and the tenacity with which it can persist throughout life are not to be underestimated.

It must be also be noted that in the case of a single traumatic episode, i.e., shock trauma (Kris, 1956), an extremely resilient child can return to the normal course of development after some disruption with no residual damage (Tyson & Tyson, 1990, p. 24). In addition, it is possible for traumatic experience to provide an impetus in some children for further development and a better adaptation than would otherwise be achieved (p. 328). The intrapsychic meaning of a traumatic experience for the individual affected, for better or for worse, is dependent on multiple factors. These include the nature and magnitude of the trauma, early-life onset, the period of development, the longevity and intensity of exposure, the situation in which it occurs, the source of the trauma, the individual's ego strength, prior traumatic experiences and the level of mastery of them, preexisting vulnerabilities, resilience and external support systems. What might be traumatic for one individual may not be for another, and what could be traumatic in one period of development for an individual might not be in another period of development (Arlow, 2006, p. 120). Anna Freud (1965) noted that development proceeds normally or not, regardless of internal or external stresses or disturbances.

The damage from trauma to the psyche of the child is due to the prolonged, repetitive traumatic situation, such as ongoing child abuse, that can have the potential to cause extensive damage to the psyche of the child, viz. Kahn's (1963) concept of cumulative trauma. This can have enduring detrimental effects on the child's development in ways that interfere with the achievement of important developmental tasks, which can lead to fixation, regression and psychopathology.

From a contemporary view of trauma and development, Bohleber (2010) believes that both the traditional psycho-economic model and the object relations model are necessary to fully comprehend and understand the psychic processes of trauma. In addition to Freud's definition of trauma as the *quantity* of excitations that flood the ego with anxiety and helplessness, the object relationship itself takes on the *quality* of trauma. In regard to the traditional model, Bohleber (2007) states that "the destructive element, the direct traumatizing force, remains something excessive, a massive surplus that ruptures the psychic structure and cannot be bound through meaning" (p. 340). In the object relations model of trauma, among all of the circumstances in which trauma can occur—e.g., sexual abuse, extreme emotional neglect, separation trauma, attachment trauma, cumulative trauma, etc.—intrafamilial trauma can be among the most devastating. "The most intensely pathogenic element is mistreatment or abuse by the person whose protection and care is actually needed" (Bohleber, 2017, pp. 3–4). Such experiences can have a profound and life-long impact on the child, unlike in the case of adult-onset trauma. Children who are exposed to prolonged, unmanageable stress, especially at the hands of a parent, are highly vulnerable to being impaired in their ability to successfully accomplish the tasks of the early stages of development.

It is also necessary to consider that trauma itself is not the only consideration in evaluating clinical cases involving trauma of any kind. It is a common view that intrapsychic conflict may already exist prior to the traumatic event(s) (see Spivak, this volume). Busch notes that it is important to consider an integrated perspective between early trauma and intrapsychic conflict. He says that intrapsychic conflict can also be a *result* of early traumatic experience. He cites Smith's (2003) view that there are various ways to consider conflict: "it is not only the trauma itself that remains traumatic. Inevitably, the *feelings and fantasies that the trauma stimulates* become part of a dangerous intrapsychic field. *In this way, a trauma also becomes part of an intrapsychic conflict*" (Busch, 2005, pp. 27–28, italics in original).

Sugarman (2008) states that in evaluating trauma one must consider that neither the external environment nor the internal world alone is thought to cause any single mental phenomenon. He argues against a relational treatment approach that excludes the perspective of preexisting internal conflict. He "assumes that trauma, even childhood trauma, is usually experienced and processed by an already more-or-less structured mind that will define what is traumatic, as well as attempt to make sense of it" (p. 801; see also Sugarman, 2018). Like Busch, he also finds that feelings and fantasies generated by the trauma become components of intrapsychic conflict and compromise formation.

Traumatic memories

In order to have a thorough consideration of the significant aspects of trauma, it is important to consider the role of traumatic memories. This is because of the function of memory in the controversy over the etiological role of trauma in pathogenesis. In Gaensbauer's description of traumatic memories, he states that:

> memory researchers have conceptualized two functionally distinct systems of memory: procedural, implicit, or early memory and declarative, explicit, or late memory…Procedural or implicit knowledge refers to the largely unconscious, automatically operating memory systems related to behavioral, emotional, and sensory experience (1995, p. 124).

These memories may be manifested in certain aspects of the transference, and in traumatic triggers that can be experienced in somatic sensations, traumatic dreams and intense affective states with no content. They inevitably appear to go back directly to the early trauma, as in the case of states of dissociation (see Diamond, this volume). "Declarative or explicit memory refers to knowledge that is conscious, can be recalled as coming from the past and can be communicated to others directly" (Gaensbauer, 1995, p. 124), such as autobiographical memory, which is the ability to represent oneself as having participated in a particular activity at a particular time and place in the past.

When discussing the nature of explicit memories in regard to trauma, Bohleber goes on to say that, based on recent studies in cognitive science, "memories of acutely and stressful traumatic events are predominantly highly detailed, extremely constant and, as far as can be judged, also relatively reliable" (2007, p. 337; also Bohleber, 2010); that is, they constitute a special set of experiences that are generally preserved in the particulars and with great precision over a long period. This is particularly significant because it contradicts the assertion by some that all childhood traumas originate from the outside, e.g., from traumatogenic relationships with important early objects, with no contribution from inside the mind of the child. Also, relational and self psychological analysts, as well as some contemporary Kleinians, tend to minimize the importance of internal conflict. A central feature of this position is that memories of the trauma are stored in implicit, non-declarative memory systems which are accessible to treatment only through reexperiencing the trauma through the analytic relationship (Sugerman, 2008). This has distinctive implications for the treatment approach. In contrast to an either/or position, Gaensbauer (1995) reports that research on preverbal traumas shows that they are remembered both procedurally and declaratively.

Case presentation

When Mr. B began analysis he had been desperately unhappy for most of his life. He appeared to be in the grip of a disorganized, primitive and prepsychotic state of mind. He was alienated from the outside world around him, including his family. He was suspicious of others, socially isolated and terrified of his own inner demons, as well as the outer forces which he feared could turn against him at any time.

Mr. B felt different from other "normal" people, toward whom he had festering feelings of envy, spite and hatred, as well as fantasies of revenge for his unfair lot in life. In turn, this state of his internal world caused him to have pervasive feelings of self-hatred, shame, guilt and paranoia, with fears of retaliation against him and intense anxiety. He felt that people could see all of these contents of his internal world. This made him an "open book".

This prism through which Mr. B viewed himself functioned as a prison itself, isolating him from other people as well as from educational and job opportunities. His view of himself was that he had been born bad and was destined to live out his life in continuous misery. It stemmed from the fact that he had been verbally and emotionally abused by his father from around the age of two years to the age of ten, at which time his parents separated. Prior to that time, it appeared that he had been well cared for by his mother and his grandmother up to the age of two, and seemed to have had sufficient nurturing to provide a secure attachment and normal development. Subsequent to this, Mr. B had some early memories of his father yelling at him in a threatening way, as well as some other incidences, but they did not seem to have had a traumatic effect.

However, it was the memory of a particular event around the age of four that Mr. B considers to be a defining moment in his history of trauma. It had an indelible effect on him. He vividly remembers that he was with both of his parents on their bed, mother in her nightgown and father shirtless. He observed them engaged in a kind of light erotic foreplay, "kidding around about 'titties'". He remembers being curious, wanting to be included, and feeling it would be natural for him to join in, yet also feeling tentative about it. At a certain point, he reached out and touched his mother's breast. Instantly, his father exploded at him. He recounted the shock of his father's reaction. It stunned him and catapulted him into a state of terror, helplessness and utter confusion.

At the time, Mr. B had no awareness that his father's aggressive behavior toward him was abusive. Rather, he believed that he deserved it because of his feeling that he was inherently bad and that he had been born that way. As a result of this distorted perception of himself, he had long-standing feelings of self-blame and self-hatred. He also remembered another incident that occurred shortly thereafter. His mother had left him in the care of his father as she was about to go out. When he began to cry at being left alone with his father, he remembers his father "putting his fist in my face and yelling, 'I'll give you something to cry about!' That meant that I couldn't show my feelings, and I haven't cried since." While these memories stand out in Mr. B's mind, he recounted a number of other instances when his father's unpredictable eruptions of anger left him in a daily state of dread. This constituted a state of cumulative trauma that lasted for eight years.

Returning to the issue of memory, the distinction between implicit and explicit memory is important because each mode is manifested in different ways, which has different implications for treatment. There is evidence of both memory functions in Mr. B's case. Implicit memory is evident when trauma gets triggered in the transference or by dreams, or by seemingly ordinary events like illness or car trouble. These reactions are dissociated recapitulations of the trauma from the past. However, most of Mr. B's memories are explicit. Bohleber's (2007) view of explicit, declarative memory, described above, is most useful in understanding the traumatized state of his mind growing up. Mr. B's memories are quite explicit. That Mr. B's memories of his father's abuse were real has been objectively verified. Earlier indications of paternal abuse were confirmed by his grandmother, who told him that when he was younger, his father had put his hands on a hot heater "to teach him a lesson". He also remembers his aunt saying to his father, "Why do you treat him that way?", to which his father responded, "He has to learn!" There is another memory of a shopper in the market who reprimanded Mr. B's father for the way he was treating his son. After they left, his father warned him, "If you tell your mother about this, I'll break your arm." Later, when Mr. B was older, after his parents had divorced and his father had remarried, he observed that his father treated his step-children the same way that he had treated him. Some of Mr. B's memories may have been modified somewhat over time, but they are sufficiently detailed that they undoubtedly have authenticity. However, it is feasible that they also serve a screen memory function in representing other incidences of abuse that he does not remember (Freud, 1951, pp. 26–27).

The memory of the primal scene event is the keystone of all of the years that Mr. B endured his father's abuse. It has iconic significance. The preserved details of the memory of the trauma appear to authenticate that the abuse was real (Bohleber, 2007), and launched the revised narrative of his experience once he was able to see the reality through the analysis. But up to this point Mr. B still was not aware that he had been abused, or that it was traumatic. And he could not yet tolerate becoming aware. That was yet to come. He continued to hold on to his lifelong belief that his internal reality as he perceived it to be the way things were, that he was treated the way he was because there was something wrong with him. His only conclusion was that it must be that he was inherently "bad". At the same time, the event has particular significance in terms of the oedipal implications of Mr. B's own internal state of mind, in conjunction with his father's abusive behavior toward him, which will be discussed later.

The negative feelings that surfaced in Mr. B's distorted fantasies of the meaning of his experience of abuse were expressed in the negative transference by a preponderance of projection, projective identification and splitting which were manifested in the profile given in the beginning of the case presentation. It was a very long struggle before he could begin to feel sufficient emotional and relational security to be open to my interpretations. Despite his explicit memories, he was dissociated from the reality of the abuse and the cumulative trauma that he had sustained in conjunction with it. This is an example of what Person and Klar (1994) refer to as vertical splitting in isolating traumatic experience, rather than horizontal splitting that occurs with the repression of fantasy content associated with internal conflict, which was also present in terms of deeper oedipal conflicts. It appeared to be in the service of self-preservation. It was a remnant of the bind that Mr. B was in as a child, unable to survive without his parents whom he needed and loved. Any acknowledgment of the fact of the abuse would have made his living situation untenable. It also became a prominent part of his internal reality.

In the transference, I became the demanding, punitive, abusive father who would come down on Mr. B and destroy him in an instant. At a deeper level, I was also the castrating father of the oedipal situation. As a result, he had great difficulty trusting me, feeling suspicious, wary of being controlled, extremely sensitive to my criticism, and frightened of his own hateful and spiteful feelings toward me. He was enraged much of the time for what he felt to be my unattainable expectations, even his interpretation of my suggestion to him to "say whatever comes to mind", which was an example of what he called my "imperatives". This was an inevitable enactment of his feeling in the familiar bind of being pressed to reveal all of his feelings of hatred, fantasies of revenge, sadism and even murder, on the one hand—while to express them, on the other hand, would expose and confirm the innate badness that he felt about himself, and would subject him to unbearable shame and humiliation. To add to this, it came out much later that he was also having extremely conflicted homosexual fantasies about me, or of being seduced by me. I understood this as stemming in part from the time during his adolescence when, feeling small and inferior, he idealized other boys whom he admired. It seemed to be an attempt to identify with them in order to consolidate his own masculine identity (Blos, 1972). His homosexual fantasies could also provide an alternative when confronted with the impossibility of getting past the incest barrier in his struggle with relationships with women. Understandably, he questioned whether or not he was gay. This was a highly delicate area that required extreme tact on my part, one that would have to wait for his readiness to address at a later time. His openness about this was as far as he could go.

At the same time, Mr. B clung desperately to the hope of getting my help. His worst fear was that I would retaliate against him and banish him from the analysis, in which case all would be lost. The strain was palpable for both of us. This early period can be seen as comparable to Searles' postulation of the autistic phase in the development of the patient-analyst mode of relatedness. According to Searles (1973, p. 247), the autistic phase is a necessary one that lasts for a protracted period of time in the transition to what he calls the therapeutic symbiosis phase, the phase in which the analyst can finally find it feasible to begin to make effective interpretations. While it is common for the analyst to feel useless and incompetent, among other things, during this time, its purpose is the establishment of reliability through the analyst's maintenance of the several aspects of the frame, the provision of an extended protected environment and the constancy of the relationship (pp. 257–258). This was a time during which I could feel Mr. B's murderous rage and terror within the silence, which he was conscious of but couldn't say. This would last for months. I also felt the helplessness of the same bind that he felt he was in, paralyzed from doing anything other than remaining constant and available, to provide an environment in which he could develop a sense of reliability in which to extricate himself and begin to find his own voice separate from me. I came to understand this from several early encounters when I mistakenly tried to address his silence, which would provoke the impasse of rage and fear. It was necessary for me to bear the strain and contain his and my own discomfort and anxiety, part of the ongoing enactment.

During a serious crisis in the transference relationship, Mr. B felt that his only choice was to capitulate to his perceptions of my imperatives or to leave the analysis, neither of which was acceptable to him. Through this painful struggle he was able to spontaneously discover his own innate capacity for introspection. This was an example of the early ego strength that had been dissociated and preserved in his psyche for years. It was a significant transition. This realization enabled him to detach himself from my prescriptive rules enough to finally begin to free associate according to his own sense of agency. He began to let go and talk more freely about his own feelings, thoughts and observations, somewhat independent of my expectations, while remaining extremely wary of potential criticism from me. Still, it was a critical turning point in the analysis which relieved the tremendous strain that had existed between us for what felt like an interminable time.

Eventually, Mr. B. was able to begin to accept my interpretation of the reality of the abuse to which he had been subjected. Later, he could also recognize that it had been traumatic for most of his childhood. This was the beginning of the revised narrative of his experience based on the external reality of his father's abuse. His childhood interpretation that he was inherently bad had enabled him to preserve the goodness of his parents, whom he loved and needed, in order to survive (Fairbairn, 1952, in terms of the tenacity of the patient's internal closed world). It was still extremely difficult for him to relinquish his position as the one to blame. Mr. B gradually came to grasp the reality of his father's abusive behavior toward him and the damage that it had caused psychically, so that he could also begin to attribute it to its proper source, rather than to his innate badness. He also saw how profoundly his original interpretation had affected his view of himself and his relationship to others. He began to cultivate his capacity for self-reflection and introspection. This enabled him to begin to integrate the disturbing feelings triggered by the trauma, initiating a process of working though. Now, he was more able to rely on existing, or to develop new, ego strengths which enhanced his ability to regulate his feelings, deal with other people more effectively and conduct himself generally. Over time, his life became significantly improved and fairly stable.

The black hole: the trauma of abuse

It became apparent very early that Mr. B was quite intelligent, highly imaginative and verbally articulate. He had always had a unique capacity to express himself. Some time after he became aware that his father's harsh treatment of him was abusive, he happened upon Stephen Hawking's book *A Brief History of Time: From the Big Bang to Black Holes* (1988). From his interpretation of Hawking's description of the creation of a black hole from the massive collapse of a dying star in which objects get hopelessly sucked and trapped, he gleaned a parallel between what happens astrologically and what he had internalized as a result of the abuse. The black hole became a particularly idiosyncratic metaphor for all of the manifestations of the damage to his psyche that he had internalized. His usurpation of the concept of the "black hole" was coincidental to frequent references to it in the psychoanalytic literature to designate a feature of trauma (Eshel, 1998; Grotstein, 1990, and others). Everything that he experienced was drawn into the black hole of his internal world. There was no escape, there was no hope. After that, it was just a short step from the metaphor of the black hole to the recognition that the abuse he had sustained had also been traumatic.

From then on, Mr. B began to elaborate on the multiple aspects of the abuse and to recognize the damaging effects it had inflicted on him. He moved from his former dissociated primitive thinking to a developing capacity for symbolization through the use of words to articulate a more accurate and meaningful understanding of his experience. This is an example of what Brenner (2014) describes as the entry into the role of symbolization in the transformation of the unarticulated and unspeakable into the articulation of experience through the use of words. The creation of the metaphor of the black hole itself was an early example of this development in the analysis.

As a result, Mr. B began to work to correct the distorted perceptions of his experience and its damaging aspects. As long as he could remember, he had felt that he was to blame. The black hole came to represent the container of all of the festering feelings of envy, spite and hate that he loathed in himself, as well as the fears of exposure and reprisal that would comprise a "fate worse than death". Now he started to realize that he had taken all the blame for his father's treatment of him. After all, part of the abuse was that his father *was*, in fact, blaming him. Now, Mr. B could say, "It wasn't me, it was my own father. He was supposed to be loving and protective of me, not some stranger whom I didn't know, who treated me that way." The combination of the fact that it was his own father, his father's large size and authority over him, in comparison to his small size and weakness, the force of his father's loud tone of voice, "always yelling", his profanity, his verbal threats—for example, "I'll give you something to cry about"—all magnified Mr. B's reactions and were a daily presence in his mind. This was coupled with the sense of betrayal and disillusionment that he felt that his mother didn't intervene to protect him. Consider Kahn's idea of the mother's function as a protective shield (1963): "As a result, I couldn't trust her either."

Mr. B's identifications with his father were mixed. There were signs of some healthy identifications in his idealization of things about his father that he was proud of. But they were subverted by his father's abuse and his fear and hatred of him, and he rejected them. Instead, the damage from the abuse led to his identification with his father as the aggressor as a defense (Freud, 1936). It was out of this identification that he created the black hole to contain all of the negative introjects of his father's abuse. He said:

> I identified with Dad in a bad way. "If you can't beat 'em, join 'em." I internalized whatever it was that made him treat me the way he did; all the hatred and negative feeling that I felt from him. I did him one better! I turned them on myself. That was the real damage! I became a clone of Dad and it made me despise myself.

Shengold (1989) says that among the damages from abuse, the child takes over all the feelings of guilt and shame that the parent should have, which can result in a sadistic superego and a masochistic ego. This was the case with Mr. B., who took all of the despicable things about his father that he had internalized and turned them against himself and into the contents of the black hole. This was a measure of the extent of the trauma to which Mr. B was subjected.

In his work with a spectrum of patients, Busch (2005, p. 28) states that he has tended "to work *first* with implications of interferences in narcissistic development" (e.g., abuse), while being aware of guilt-arousing feelings of conflict (oedipal) before directly raising them. Most of Mr. B's lengthy analysis to this point concentrated on the abuse and its traumatic effects. His acknowledgment of the reality of his experience of abuse and its traumatic impact and his considerable insight into the distorted logic that he had used to rationalize the abuse yielded significant results. Included were his recognition of the new external and internal reality, the resurgence of his earlier rudimentary ego strengths (affect regulation, judgment, impulse control, object constancy) and the integration of the splits from his all or nothing, good or bad thinking into an appreciation of the complexities involved in all aspects of self and others, as well as relationships. Mr. B began to feel a stronger sense of continuity, constancy and wholeness within himself, rather than the fragmented sense that he had felt for most of his life. He also acquired newfound insight into, and empathy for, other people different from himself, as well as a growing sense of trust in others. Finally, he achieved a growing sense of agency, with the ability to stand up for himself to others, including his father.

The last frontier: the oedipal phase

The significance of the oedipal phase and the development of oedipal object relations and sexuality itself has receded in the psychoanalytic literature in recent decades with the emerging emphasis on earlier stages of psychic life. However, it is still considered to be a crucial stage of psychosexual development, encompassing virtually all of the evolving psychological functions of the previous phase, when the forces of sexuality and aggression are tamed, the superego is formed and feelings of guilt emerge (Loewald, 1979; Gilmore & Meersand, 2014). In contemporary psychoanalysis, the importance of the oedipal phase goes beyond Freud's theory of the oedipal drama of the male child's incestuous desires for the mother, murderous fantasies toward the father and fears of castration. In addition to the transformation of the mother–child dyad into triadic relationships, the presence of new and complicated conscious and unconscious fantasies, the influences of early gender identifications and the development of the superego, the oedipal phase includes the development of a myriad other capacities. They include, but are not limited to, language development, the development of cognition and symbolization, and an early capacity for mentalization. Mentalization constitutes the regulation and organization of emotional life, i.e., the ability to reflect on the mental life of one's own and others, which grows mostly out of the child's primary object relationships. It involves both self-reflective and interpersonal components (Fonagy & Target, 2003).

In the analysis of Mr. B, oedipal manifestations were always mixed in with his associations of the trauma of the abuse. But due to his preoccupation with the abuse, they weren't available for analysis. However, as the effects of the damage from the abuse subsided and insight and growth continued to develop, concerns of sexuality, intimacy and love began to emerge and become more prominent. As a result, oedipal issues started to become more accessible. He began to shift to his relationships with women and his desire to have a loving sexual relationship with one. He had had relationships with women when he was younger, but he had been unable to sustain a long-term, emotionally intimate sexual relationship with any of them.

In addition, Mr. B was troubled by intrusive images of his mother when he was having sex with women, which would render him impotent. He remembers having incestuous fantasies as a child, which were instigated by seeing his mother walking around the house half-naked. He also revealed an incident, at age eight, of being aroused and having extremely confused and conflicted feelings of guilt, shame and inadequacy when his mother coaxed him into massaging her feet and legs, up to her thighs, after a long day at work. This was coupled with the conscious fear that his father would suddenly appear and smash him down.

Mr. B refers to the focus on his sexuality and his relationships with women as the "last frontier". The last frontier represents the last to be settled, explored or developed in a country or region, as well as the extreme limit of understanding or achievement in a particular area. It is striking that the current view of the "final frontier" made popular by the opening narration of the series *Star Trek* should correspond to the similar metaphor relating to the outer space of the black hole. But, the metaphor of the black hole symbolizes loss and hopelessness, while the last frontier connotes exploration and hope for the future.

For Mr. B, the last frontier represents the complexity of his sexuality and his struggles in his relationships with women. His heightened awareness of his mother, exacerbated by the inappropriate sexually charged exposure by his parents in the primal scene situation, the seductive nakedness of his mother and the foot massaging incident, all contributed to his incestuous fantasies and caused great anxiety in him. The fantasies of his mother, combined with the fear of his father, are fused with other women and the threat of being attacked and destroyed by another man if he becomes intimate with them. He also feels the inability to compete with other men, feeling small, weak and inadequate in comparison with them. This is evidence of the interruption in his oedipal development, which he characterized as "small boy, small penis". This was partly the result of Mr. B's feeling of being "smashed down" by his father's abuse; but it also seems to due to his oedipal victory over his father in the competition for his mother. It left him with considerable castration anxiety. After all, his mother divorced his father, while he stayed. He won a mother whom he couldn't satisfy, and he rejected a father from whom he could derive his own masculine identity and strength. This was a significant aspect of his unresolved Oedipus complex. This constituted a huge barrier to the achievement of his wish to have an integrated intimate, emotional and sexual relationship with a woman. This was the challenge of the last frontier.

.By the age of four, when the primal scene event occurred, Mr. B would have achieved some level of ego development that allowed him to reality test, to have some level of judgment and impulse control, and to differentiate internal from external, self from other, and between thoughts, feelings and behavior. Even though these strengths were subverted and seemed to be lost due to the severe regressive effect of the abuse, they remained partially intact and occasionally surfaced in his conscious mind. Consider Sugarman's (2008) position about an already structured mind, referenced in the memory section above. Oedipal fantasies would also undoubtedly have been active in his mind. Tyson & Tyson (1990) speak about developmental interferences: "at the peak of the infantile genital phase, the child may interpret [them] as punishment for oedipal wishes, which may exacerbate castration anxiety" (p. 28). Given his intelligence, it is also feasible that he had a precocious mind, which may account for his awareness of his feelings in the situation as part of the freeze in his memory as an aspect of the trauma. It seemed likely that the magnitude of the impact of the attacks on him by his father was fueled by his own oedipal fantasies, which he would have felt as quite dangerous and which added to the trauma. While his conscious emphasis was on his father's abuse and his perception of his mother's collusion with it, unconsciously this was conflated with his oedipal conflicts. For example, in the context of speaking about the abuse he revealed that he remembered fantasizing consciously about wishing his father dead, "because he was blocking me from Mom. I wanted him out of the way. But then I thought, He's my father. I shouldn't feel that way. It confirms that I must be bad." In addition to feeling guilty for wishing his father dead, he was also afraid that his father could see what was in his mind, and would become enraged and kill him.

Referring to the primal scene incident, Mr. B said,

> It hit me like the Big Bang! In an instant, my whole world was shattered. If I'm prohibited from touching Mom and being intimate with her like I was before, that meant that I couldn't love her either because Dad would smash me down.

This was a metastatic change. Later, it also meant that he couldn't love any other woman either, because some surrogate of Dad would appear and destroy him. These others became transference figures in his mind in his struggle to have a satisfying whole relationship with a woman. "If I can't love Mom, I can't love any other woman either. And because Mom didn't protect me from him, it's fused with my feelings about other women. I can't trust them either." At the same time, he relied on his mother for her love and protection. She was his refuge. "I always knew that she loved me in spite of the betrayal." However, the incestuous fantasies remained active, and interfered with his ability to feel like his own man and to relate to women independently of his attachment to his mother. Among other things, they hindered him in this necessary struggle to separate from her (Diamond, 2006).

Up to this point, Mr. B still viewed himself as an innocent victim of the abuse. Despite blaming himself for his father's abusive behavior, he still had no sense of agency or responsibility for his own fantasies or actions. Touching his mother's breast was purely a residue of having been an infant at the breast. He had no conscious awareness of any hint of sexuality, or even of sensuality. His focus was still on the abuse. However, the sexual content of what Mr. B was now talking about made the connection to oedipal issues just a step away in his preconscious mind. In brief spurts, he began to recall the feelings that he had felt while his parents were playing in the primal scene. Later, he remembered noticing that his mother was relating to his father in a way that he hadn't been aware of before, a way that made him feel excluded from what was going on between them. He needed reassurance that his relationship with her had remained intact from what it had always been before. While he had the urge to join in, he also felt hesitant before touching her breast, questioning whether he should, yet he reached for it anyway. With the purpose of highlighting his oedipal conflicts over the abuse and to link them, I suggested that he might consider that, in addition to his father's threats, part of the intensity of his reaction to his father's abusive attack was fueled by his preexisting desire to have his mother all to himself, his wish to get rid of his father and his fear of his father's retaliation. He could begin to make use of this awareness and to link the abuse and his sexuality in a way that broadened his understanding of his childhood situation. It opened him up to begin to take ownership in the oedipal drama as an antidote to the victim stance that he'd taken in life as a result of being abused.

Since then, the perception of me that Mr. B had in the transference has begun to change. As his castration fears and feelings of inferiority and intimidation in relation to me continue to linger, he is also beginning to see me as a more benign and benevolent figure in his life. As a result, he is able to talk more openly about feelings and fantasies toward me, including homosexual conflicts. I still don't dare to comment for concern that I will derail him and risk provoking a severe negative transference reaction which could seriously disrupt the analysis. I take the stance of relying on his own self-reflective tendencies and to wait for him to reach a point where he can tolerate an interpretation about his castration fears. Mr. B has softened in his attitude toward his father as well, recalling loving things that his father did, like caring for him when he was sick and teaching him how to surf and fish. For example, he remembered a time when his father took him hiking and seemed to transform into a different person. He saw his father being sensitive to the sights and smells of nature, smelling the leaves from the trees and sharing his experience of their being together.

For some time now, Mr. B has begun to speak more often about his sense of his own manhood, his sexuality and the love he has felt for the opposite sex all his life. He has begun to flirt openly with some of the women he works with, and to share some of the active sexual fantasies that he has about them with me, all within appropriate bounds. He feels a significant freedom from his inhibitions and is more able to behave spontaneously and unselfconsciously with them. This is a continuation of the development that had been interrupted so many years ago, evidence of a growing sense of "grown man, grown penis".

Conclusion

In today's therapeutic climate, there has been an explosion of articles, books and workshops on trauma. Within this phenomenon, a polarization of views among analysts about the etiological role of trauma on a range of mental disturbances, and the clinical implications that follow, has taken place, as referred to above (Busch, 2005; Bohleber, 2007; Sugarman, 2008; Spivak, this volume).

The dichotomy is between those more traditional analysts who believe that preexisting intrapsychic conflict is reflected in the individual's response to trauma as well as on the development of conflict subsequent to the trauma and those relational analysts and others who emphasize the role of external reality, especially relationships with important early objects, as the cause of trauma. In this latter view, internal mental structures are deemphasized as being significant causative factors.

In terms of treatment, traditional analysts emphasize the importance of addressing internal conflicts, both preexisting and those inherent to the trauma. This includes unconscious feelings and fantasies created by the trauma and defenses against them, with the goal of promoting conscious awareness toward insight and self-understanding in working through all of the aspects of the trauma. Remembering, reconstruction and interpretation are central factors in this approach.

Others, working with trauma alone, focus on the analytic relationship with close attunement to the feeling and emotional state of the patient. The patient's life history and factual memories are set aside in favor of a focus on implicit or procedural memories of trauma which are enacted, reexperienced and modified through the transference relationship with the analyst.

The authors cited above all consider both views of trauma to be important. They believe that the analyst's empathic attunement for the purpose of creating an atmosphere of safety is important in the treatment of trauma, and that external contributants to the trauma and the importance of object relationships must be considered as well. Yet, given their position that preexisting conflict is present in the trauma, as well as conflicts created by the trauma, a more traditional approach that considers both trauma and intrapsychic conflict, can be more effective. Sugarman (2008) states that "analysts who emphasize the importance of conflict in trauma … see [it] as accessible to verbal self-reflective analysis, in the same manner as other unknown thoughts, feelings, and experiences are" (p. 802).

Mr. B's focus on the abuse and the damage to his psyche exemplifies the danger of external factors being the only objective of treatment. This approach would have been at the expense of attending to his preexisting oedipal conflicts, conflicts which were present from the beginning. There was ample evidence of an unresolved Oedipus complex which, combined with the effects of his father's abuse, radically affected the psychic organization of his mind. His oedipal conflicts contributed to, and were exacerbated by, the trauma of the abuse. This supports the thesis that both external events and internal reality are inextricably bound in both directions in navigating the oedipal situation. Therefore, it has been necessary to work with both, each in conjunction with the other, in order to achieve the goal of their integration in Mr. B's mind.

In view of the multiple functions of the oedipal phase, as Blum (1991) has expressed, "Working through oedipal issues promotes maturation in general, not just sexually, which in turn strengthens a sense of self and promotes feelings of agency, self-sufficiency, competency, *and can be an antidote to abused children's process*" (italics added).

References

Ainsworth, M., Blehar, M., Waters, E. & Wall, S. (1978). *Patterns of Attachment.* Hillsdale, NJ: Lawrence Erlbaum Associates.

Arlow, J.A. (2006). Trauma and pathogenesis. *The Seduction Theory in its Second Century,* M.I. Good (ed.). Madison, CT: International Universities Press.

Blos, P. (1972). The ego ideal in adolescence. *Psychoanalytic Study of the Child*, 27: 93–97.
Blum, H.P. (1991). Sadomasochism in the psychoanalytic process, within and beyond the pleasure principle. *Journal of the American Psychoanalytic Association*, 39: 431–450.
Bohleber, W. (2007). Remembrance, trauma and cumulative memory: The battle for meaning in psychoanalysis. *International Journal of Psychoanalysis*, 88: 329–352.
Bohleber, W. (2010). *Destructiveness, Intersubjectivity and Trauma: the Identity Crisis of Modern Psychoanalysis.* London: Karnac.
Bohleber, W. (2017). New approaches to deal with trauma. Paper presented at the New Center for Psychoanalysis, Los Angeles, May 18.
Bowlby, J. (1960). Separation anxiety. *International Journal of Psychoanalysis*, 41: 89–113.
Bowlby, J. (1969). *Attachment and Loss: Attachment. Vol. 1.* New York: Basic Books.
Brenner, I. (2014). *Dark Matters: Exploring the Realm of Psychic Devastation.* London: Karnac.
Busch, F. (2005). Conflict theory/trauma theory. *Psychoanalytic Quarterly*, 74: 27–45.
Diamond, M.J. (2006). Masculinity unraveled: The roots of male gender identity and the shifting of male ego ideals throughout life. *Journal of the American Psychoanalytic Association*, 54: 1099–1130.
Eshel, O. (1998). "Black holes", deadness and existing analytically. *International Journal of Psychoanalysis*, 79: 1115–1130.
Erikson, E. (1950). *Childhood and Society.* New York: Norton.
Fairbairn, W.D.R. (1952). *Psychoanalytic Studies of the Personality.* London: Routledge.
Fonagy, P. & Target, M. (2003). *Psychoanalytic Theories: Perspectives from Developmental Pathologies.* New York & London: Routledge.
Freud, A. (1936). The ego and the mechanisms of defense. *The Writings of Anna Freud, Vol. II.* New York: International Universities Press.
Freud, A. (1951). Observations on child development. *Psychoanalytic Study of the Child*, 6: 18–30.
Freud, A. (1965). Normality and pathology in childhood: assessments of development. *The Writings of Anna Freud, Vol. VI.* New York: International Universities Press.
Freud, A. (1967). Comments on trauma. *Psychic Trauma*, S. Furst (ed.). New York: Basic Books, 235–246.
Freud, S. (1896). The aetiology of hysteria. *Standard Edition 3*: 191–221.
Freud, S. (1920). Beyond the pleasure principle. *Standard Edition 18*: 7–64.
Freud, S. (1926). Inhibitions, symptoms and anxiety. *Standard Edition 20*: 87–174.
Gaensbauer, T.J. (1995). Trauma in the preverbal period: Symptoms, memories and developmental impact. *Psychoanalytic Study of the Child*, 50: 122–149.
Galatzer-Levy, R.M. (1995). Psychoanalysis and dynamic systems theory: Prediction and self-similarity. *Journal of the American Psychoanalytic Association*, 43: 1085–1113.
Gilmore, K. (2008). Psychanalytic developmental theory: A contemporary reconsideration. *Journal of the American Psychoanalytic Association*, 56: 885–907.
Gilmore, K.J. & Meersand, P. (2014). *Development: A Psychodynamic Primer.* Washington, DC: American Psychiatric Publishing.
Grotstein, J.S. (1990). Nothingness, meaninglessness, chaos and the "black hole". *Contemporary Psychoanalysis*, 26: 257–290.
Hawking, A. (1988). *A Brief History of Time: From the Big Bang to Black Holes.* London & New York: Bantam Books.

Kahn, M. (1963). The concept of cumulative trauma. *Psychoanalytic Study of the Child*, 18: 286–306.

Kris, E. (1956). The recovery of childhood memories in psychoanalysis. *Psychoanalytic Study of the Child*, 11: 54–88.

Loewald, H.W. (1979). The waning of the Oedipus complex. *Journal of the American Psychoanalytic Association*, 27: 751–775.

Mahler, M., Pine, F. & Bergman, A. (1975). *The Psychological Birth of the Human Infant: Symbiosis and Individuation*. New York: Basic Books.

Malberg, N.T. & Mayes, L. (2015). The developmental perspective. *Handbook of Psychodynamic Approaches in Psychopathology*, P. Luyten, L.C. Mayes, P. Fonagy, M. Target, & S. Blatt (eds.). New York: Guilford Press, 47–64.

Nagera, H. (1966). *Early Childhood Disturbances, the Infantile Neurosis, and the Adulthood Disturbances: Problems of a Developmental Psychoanalytical Psychology*. New York: International Universities Press.

Person, E. & Klar, H. (1994). Establishing trauma: the difficulty distinguishing between memories and fantasies. *Journal of the American Psychoanalytic Association*, 42: 1055–1081.

Searles, H.F. (1973). Concerning therapeutic symbiosis. *Annual of Psychoanalysis*, 1: 247–262.

Shengold, L. (1989). *Soul Murder: The Effects of Child Abuse and Deprivation*. New Haven, CT: Yale University Press.

Smith, H.F. (2003). Conceptions of conflict in psychoanalytic theory and practice. *Psychoanalytic Quarterly*, 72: 49–76.

Sugarman, A. (2008). The use of play to promote insightfulness in the analysis of children suffering from cumulative trauma. *Psychoanalytic Quarterly*, 77: 799–833.

Sugarman, A. (2018). Conflict theory, nonlinear development, and mutative action with cases of cumulative trauma: Commentary of Fischer. *Journal of the American Psychoanalytic Association*, 66: 103–114.

Tyson, P. & Tyson, R.L. (1990). *Psychoanalytic Theories of Development: An Integration*. New Haven, CT: Yale University Press.

Van der Kolk, B.A. (2005). Developmental trauma disorder. *Psychiatric Annals*, 35: 401–408.

Chapter 2

The trauma of Otherness and the struggle for connection

Schizoid and sadomasochistic defenses against contact with the Other

Pamela Dirham

Introduction

In this chapter I am going to discuss the analysis of a patient for whom contact with the Other was experienced as an existential threat that must be warded off at all costs. Due to severe early maternal deprivation, the patient, whom I will call Jack, developed a psychic structure of an omnipotent, closed schizoid system (Fairbairn, 1952). As Ogden (2010) describes it,

> Fairbairn's conception of early psychic development is a trauma theory in which the infant, to varying degrees, is traumatized by his realistic perception that he is fully dependent on a mother whose capacity to love him has passed its breaking point. (p. 91)

These "varying degrees" of trauma produce feelings in the infant/child of intense humiliation, shame of having needs, worthlessness and impotence (Fairbairn, 1944). But, as Fairbairn states, there is a more catastrophic experience for the infant. He writes: "At a still deeper level (or at a still earlier stage) the child's experience is one of, so to speak, exploding ineffectively and being completely of libido. It is thus an experience of disintegration and imminent psychical death" (p. 113). The closed schizoid psychic system in which intense relationships between the (bad) mother and (bad) infant are maintained is developed, among other reasons, as a defense against the experience of total annihilation. Contact with the Other, which creates a breach into the closed psychic system, was felt by Jack as a threat to his very existence.

Fairbairn (1952) believed that sadomasochism is inherent in a closed schizoid system. He states "a relationship with a bad object can hardly escape the alternative of being either of a sadistic or of a masochistic nature" (p. 79). As we know from Freud (1915), sadism and masochism can reverse themselves and always appear together in the psyche. For Jack, sadomasochism was certainly an active force in his internal object relationships. But I believe it also served a function of warding off actual awareness of the Other, awareness of an object separate from his omnipotent subjective world. Sartre (1957), in his philosophy of the "Look of the Other", described sadomasochism as a mechanism by which a consciousness seeks to support the point of view that there is only one subjectivity, where the abuser and the abused are one entity. Sadism has as its goal the annihilation of the subjectivity of the victim (the Other). Masochism joins in, standing for the Other whose subjectivity must be destroyed. I believe that Jack employed his inevitable sadomasochism as a defense against awareness of any subjectivity other than his, thus reinforcing and protecting his closed schizoid organization.

I describe the analysis as occurring in three phases: schizoid, sadomasochistic and "sheer madness". Although dividing the analysis into distinct phases is necessarily artificial, I am doing so because I have experienced it as moving in and out of a predominantly schizoid phase, in and out of a predominantly sadomasochistic phase, and in and out of what is felt to be a phase of sheer madness. Certainly, the schizoid and sadomasochistic phases are intertwined, each providing multiple functions for the other. The phase of what I experienced as sheer madness seems related to what Balint (1968) describes as the area of the basic fault. Aside from the issue of the artificiality of this structure, I believe that our living through and surviving these phases together has enabled both of us to feel a life-enriching faith: faith in ourselves and our capacities (for Jack, the capacity to be alive); faith in each other as comrades in a desperate struggle; and faith in the process of psychoanalysis. I mean faith in the usual sense, and I also mean it to be more. Eigen (2004), in discussing the area of faith in the works of Winnicott, Lacan and Bion, describes it as a way of experiencing life that is undertaken with one's whole being. Yalom (1980) calls it whole-hearted engagement with life. Jack spoke many times about his wish for and fear of real commitment to life. His current experience of himself is one of a tentative but hopeful "diving in" to life. He, more often these days, experiences a sense of bringing his whole self to the analysis, to his private life and to his interpersonal relationships.

Family history

Jack is currently 42 years old, never married, never lived with a woman. He is the second of three children, and the only boy. During his infancy and early childhood Jack and his family lived near his mother's parents. His mother experienced severe post-partum depression with the birth of each of her children, and gave them to the care of her mother for weeks or months at a time. Jack and his family moved away from his grandparents when he was four years old.

Jack remembers the move. He was very attached to his maternal grandfather, and felt devastated at being separated from him. He remembers spending days sitting outside the new home crying. He recently learned from his parents that he cried most of the time for about 4 weeks, was unable to function normally, and had nightmares and night terrors beginning with the move and continuing until he was about ten. He remembers his father tending to him when he woke screaming. It was the most physical nurturing he remembers getting from either parent.

Jack describes his father as "mechanical" and unable to experience deep feelings. The father had difficulty relating to his wife and children, and spent most of his time out in his workshop, tinkering with some project. Jack says, "My dad could only relate to things." Jack also felt that his father lacked masculinity, was fearful and overly cautious, and was somewhat asexual.

In contrast, Jack describes his mother as powerful "in a controlling, passive-aggressive way." He experienced her as assaultive and intrusive, yet fragile and given to "falling apart at any little thing." An example he gives of her intrusiveness is that in his home no one could take a nap. Mother would wake them up, chide them for sleeping, then complain that they had left her alone and bored. His sense of her fragility includes his memory of her several brief hospitalizations for depression in the first ten years of his life. Jack says that neither of his parents ever bothered to get to know him, and still feels the pain of this non-recognition each time he visits them.

Jack began to seclude himself from family and peers around the age of 14. He was fascinated with video games and spent most of his time in his room. He chose not to attend college and lived at home until he was 28, at which time he moved to Los Angeles.

He felt his social life was lacking and his work life in the video game industry to be unsatisfactory. He began twice-weekly psychotherapy with me. During the first years of psychotherapy he wanted to "focus the therapy" on his belief that all he needed to feel good was to find "the right woman." He wanted me to help him "hone his social skills" so that he could find this woman and solve all of his problems. He gradually admitted to himself and to me that he was depressed. He realized he found no joy in life, had never really "committed to life" and, in fact, had never really felt alive. That realization terrified him. He then asked about psychoanalysis and, after some months of hesitation and discussion, began four times a week on the couch.

The schizoid phase

Jack had been an interesting and lively psychotherapy patient. Immediately upon beginning analysis, the feeling of the sessions changed. Early in the analysis he described what we were doing together as a "fee for hire" service. I was providing a service for which I was "technically" qualified, and he needed the service for help with his depression. I was taken aback by this description of what we were up to. I tried to open a discussion concerning his feelings about this viewpoint but he claimed he had none. He said that he "technically" understood that he needed the analysis but he didn't feel anything about it. His first dream in the analysis, which occurred in the first week, provided some clues about his need to keep things technical. In this dream, he found himself riding his bicycle to a session. To his horror he noticed that he was naked. He felt exposed and vulnerable. He arrived at my office/his workshop for his session and found his father there, talking to me. He noticed water coming in under the door and saw floodwaters rolling towards my office. He kept trying to get his father and me to notice the rising water, but we failed to notice it. He tried to communicate the danger to us but we were unconcerned. The floodwaters rose higher and higher, covering his body, rising up to his neck. Only his head was out of the water. He woke up in a panic. When we discussed the dream, he asked: "I'm afraid I'm going to be overwhelmed?" He asked as if to find out if that was the "right" answer. He wasn't able to have any other associations to the dream. He had no thoughts about his head remaining out of the water. However, this head, the head untouched by the floodwaters, later became the centerpiece of a recurring countertransference image that would spontaneously appear to me for several years of the analysis. Despite (and defensively, because of) the content of that first dream, Jack's early fears in the analysis concerned me exploiting him, using him for my own needs. He knew that he was a training case, and used that fact to support his conviction that I was going to use him and then discard him. He couldn't trust me. Although Jack wanted to keep the analysis a technical, fee for hire situation, he began having considerable anxiety about our relationship and what it meant for him. Would he be hurt, exploited, abused?

What emerged, often through dreams, was a set of core fears about being in a relationship. Jack feared that I would take something from him, something vital that he needed, "like you'll pull something out of my stomach." He would not be able to protect himself. He would "cave in" to my demands due to his inability to stand up for himself. He was helpless in the face of my power. He feared loss of the integrity of his sense of self, loss of control of his feelings and loss of self-esteem. Finding ways to protect himself from me was crucial. And living in his schizoid, subjective bubble provided this protection.

Jack regularly ended relationships with women due to his feelings of being controlled by them and their needs. He feared he would lose himself. He coped with this fear by finding fault with them, and ending the relationship. This pattern also played out in the transference/countertransference situation. It often took this shape: He would have an experience of intense contact and need/affection for me. These feelings of making contact with and having a need for me were usually the result of Jack feeling particularly seen and understood by me. Within a few days of this experience he would begin talking about how the analysis was going nowhere, nothing was happening, he was not getting stimulated with any fresh insights, he was thinking of quitting the analysis, and so forth. As we tried to understand these reactions to his experience of intense contact with me, what usually emerged was his feeling that he was losing himself, He felt he could trust neither himself nor me. Internally he felt "messy and out of control."

Towards the end of the first year of the analysis, as Jack began to trust me more, he began having a new experience: sinking into the couch. He called it "a delicious feeling," a state of "getting out of my head." It was blissful. He became highly attuned to the tone of my voice. He felt soothed when the tone was "right" and horribly jarred if the tone was "off". He needed me to be the environmental mother (Winnicott, 1971), tuned in, calm, soothing and reliably present. He often napped during the sessions. He was more able to associate to his dreams and other material in these "sinking into the couch" sessions. However, these blissful feelings stirred up fears of becoming "soft", fears reflected in a dream.

In the dream he was in his car (his protective shell) and the car melted due to some type of cosmic ray. He felt exposed, vulnerable and "soft" without his car, and woke up in a terror. His associations to softness included "warm," "needy," "someone's lap," "the couch," "the warmth of this office" and "crying." As we continued to discuss this fear of softness, he came to feel an intense longing for someone to hold his "soft" self, his needy self. At the same time he was extremely conflicted about being in touch with this needy self, and regularly reverted back to experiencing himself as tough and superior to needy others.

However, at around 15 months of analysis, shortly after the analysis of the "soft" dream, Jack became more and more uncomfortable. He complained that I had "made him" experience wanting intimacy, wanting love, wanting comfort. He said, "You've made me have these desires, desires that can never be met, and now I'm trapped wanting things I can never have." He said he felt worse than he ever had in his life because I had made him aware of what he wants, what he's missed out on all of his life, and what he will never have.

The moments of connection and bliss that we had experienced together were a shock and a threat to his schizoid system. He closed in on himself. This negative therapeutic reaction served a variety of functions. It returned to a feeling of safety and stability within his internal world, a world in which hatred for the needed object and hatred for the needing self predominated (Fairbairn, 1952). It cleaned up the "internal messiness" he had complained about. It warded me off by leaving me on the outside. It punished me for luring him into a relationship. It renewed and strengthened his clinging/rejecting relationship with the internal depressed, intrusive mother.

As Jack closed in on himself and retreated to the cold but safely known internal world, the analytic sessions began to feel utterly lifeless. He would begin each session reporting on his mood, describing the degrees of depression he felt. The report would be followed by one of the monologues he used to fill the time in the sessions. Typical monologues described his hopelessness, his loneliness, his inability to attract a woman that would be stimulating enough for him, his rage at himself for creating this horrible life. Any interpretation or response from me was brushed off as an intrusion into his omnipotent self-state. When I would break into the monologue to ask "How are you feeling, right here, now?" his answer was often some version of "pretty numb." But there was no interest in expanding on these feelings. He wanted to get back to his speech.

I felt as if he was trying his best to destroy the analysis, to rob it of any life or meaning. I felt he was trying to blot me out as a person. It was as if my existence was a threat to his, and I had to be killed off, one way or another. The "softness" had to be eradicated. It seemed that he was looking for a "victory through defeat" of me, of his longings to feel alive, and of the analysis (Reik, 1941). I grew bored, angry, stultified, dead. I made the (silent) interpretation that he had succeeded in turning me into the lifeless mother. Would I be trapped in this role with him forever? Whenever I tried to say something of this kind to him he would brush me away and continue his monologue. Months and months of these dead and deadly sessions would go by without a breath of life. During one of his long, intellectualized sterile rambles I had a spontaneous fantasy. I imagined holding a samurai sword in my hands and bringing it down hard across his neck, beheading him. I imagined the head falling off the couch and rolling across the floor of my office. I felt happy. I felt alive. I came to enjoy the spontaneous appearance of this fantasy. For reasons that I did not understand then, it gave me hope.

I've come to see the multilayered meanings in this countertransference fantasy, but at first I understood it as my wish to "get him out of his head". I remembered that first dream, where the rushing floodwaters covered his body but left his head intact. I wondered if the waters were the "waters of life", that is, feelings. In the dream the waters covered his body, and, in fact, Jack experienced emotions mainly through his body. He would say "I must be anxious, my stomach is queasy" or "I might have been sad because my body had no energy."

Like me with my samurai fantasy, Jack, too, had an (unconscious) technique for restoring life into himself, me and the sessions. He would attempt to "pin me down" by insisting that I answer a theoretical question or that I provide personal information. I often experienced this behavior as a "wrestling match" with sexual overtones, ending in some kind of climax, which often took the form of an experience of intense anger at me for not answering his specific question. Some of these "wrestling matches" were more productive than others. During the unproductive ones I felt like he was experiencing me as an internal masturbatory object, hoping for whatever excitement he could create for himself. I was treated as a subjective object (Winnicott, 1971) existing in his internal world, and from whom he could get no real sustenance. I believe that since he could get no sustenance from me as his subjective object, he was determined to "get something from me" in these sessions. During the more productive "wrestling matches" he would start out using me in this way but end up relating to me as a real person, outside of his personal omnipotence. He was able to use me as his analyst and receive the "softness" he craved. He experienced these moments of climax/catharsis ending in "softness" as nourishment. After sessions such as these he would often describe himself as "satiated." The following is an excerpt from a session in which the "wrestling match" moved out of its usual controlled schizoid/masturbatory frame and into something messier, more chaotic and more productive.

The day before this session he had expressed, briefly and without feeling, his sense that he might need me and desire me.

He says, "I feel terrible, I am extremely depressed, everything is hopeless, what's the point, it's the same old thing, nothing ever changes, I'll be alone and suffering the rest of my life, why live like this ...?"

I comment on the shift from yesterday when he was feeling better.

He says, "It's always this way, I always end up getting depressed again, it's hopeless, nothing ever changes."

I ask when these feelings started.

He says, "This morning." Then he's quiet, a stubborn quiet.

I wait.

He says, "I looked in the mirror today and I saw how old and ugly and bitter I look and I thought who is going to want me, how am I ever going to get my needs met?" (a familiar monologue, but today with some feeling).

I comment on how much he is attacking himself today.

He agrees.

I link his self-attacks today to his experience of needing me and desiring me yesterday.

He says, dismissively, "That could be the case, I don't know how these things work, I just know that I always end up depressed."

I ask, "I wonder if you want to get some distance from me today?"

He says, "Technically, maybe." Then after a long pause he says, "How can you tell if a patient is making progress?"

I am a little thrown off by this and I say, "What are you asking?"

He says, "There must be some technical markers that show a patient is getting better, so what are they?"

I believe that he is focusing on this technical question to avoid talking about his self-attacks after feeling his need of and desire for me. I say something to that effect.

He says, "Yeah, maybe, but do you think I am making progress and what do you use to measure that progress?"

I'm starting to feel very confused, off balance. I decide to repeat my previous interpretation.

He says, "You are being evasive, you're often evasive when I ask you a question (in a very complaining voice) and I think you are being evasive now. Do you think I am making progress?"

I feel angry now. He is pushing me around and I don't like it. I (unconsciously) decide to "throw my weight around" by just repeating the previous interpretation.

He seems to be getting anxious, not angry, when he says, "What are you talking about? And why won't you just answer the question?"

I think to myself that this isn't the usual "wrestling match". Something is happening between us that is taking on a desperate feeling. I say something like "There's a desperate feeling to your question."

He says, "I can't understand what you are saying. (He looks to be in real distress.) Can you repeat it? Can you repeat the question? Is there a question or are you just stating something?"

I say, "Something is happening in here right now and you can't understand what I'm saying."

He started crying and the crying became sobs. He cried for a while and then said, "I feel very small, I feel like a baby, (he cries harder) and I feel you are looking at me in the crib and I can't understand what you are saying but you are there and you are looking at me" (he cries harder). I make sympathetic noises and I feel really moved and my eyes are a little wet as he sobs and sobs. He slowly settles down and naps for a minute. Then the session is over.

This productive "wrestling match" enlivened the analysis for a while. Jack was able to associate to his experience in the session. His association to the importance of seeing me looking at him as he lay in the crib was linked directly to his desperate need to be seen. As we explored these feelings further, it became clear that he experienced feeling anonymous as an unbearable narcissistic injury. I made the interpretation that the intensity of his feelings about being anonymous might be linked with the terrifying feelings he had when, as an infant and child, he did not feel seen or known by either of his parents, and particularly by his mother. At this point in the session he became very tearful. After a while he said that he did not know why he was crying but it felt good in a weird way. We again, if only briefly, felt genuine contact and connection. I noted how often these "productive" wrestling matches happened when he provoked me to anger, thus rousing me from my deadness and stupor. I wondered in what ways he had attempted to provoke his mother into aliveness, and how catastrophic it must have felt to be unable to bring her to life.

Each time we made contact there existed a window of time for us to think together about the meanings of his fears and longings. We came to feel great compassion for the lonely, needy baby who experienced his mother as dead and lifeless, often absent, and absent even when present. In doing so, Jack's attitude towards his needs for "softness" softened. He began creating a warm, comfortable living space for himself. He took in two stray cats and adopted a dog. He expanded his friendship network and was less lonely.

Despite these internal and external changes, Jack's relationships with others were mainly experienced through his schizoid system. Others remained "bundles of projections" (Winnicott, 1971) with whom he played out his internal object relationships. His fears of being engulfed by, controlled by and eventually destroyed by others (especially women) remained. This showed itself most clearly in his relationship to sex and sexuality. Jack saw himself as "highly sexual" and described himself that way many times during the analysis. He bitterly obsessed on the "irony" that although he was highly sexual, he rarely had the opportunity to have sex. Jack appeared to experience neither embarrassment nor excitement, neither guilt nor shame, when he described his sexual fantasies or sexual activities to me.

Because Jack felt so comfortable telling me about his sexual fantasies and activities, we were able to discern several patterns that greatly surprised him. One thing we discovered was that, although he obsessed about sex and his lack of it, when he actually had intercourse with a woman he would think, during the sex act, "What was all that craving about … this is really no big deal." He would find himself "going through the motions" and hoping it would be over soon. He was rarely able to ejaculate. When he got a steady girlfriend that he was very fond of, he found himself in the same position—going through the motions. He and I puzzled over this situation but came to no conclusions. Then one day he came to the session looking anxious. He began reporting the previous night's sexual activity with his girlfriend. He told his story: During sex with his girlfriend, she began having an intense orgasm, seemingly lost in an ecstatic experience. A terrible sensation of falling came over him. He had an intense fear that he was going to fall into her vagina and be swallowed up. He began having an anxiety attack but successfully hid it from his girlfriend. In the session Jack made the interpretation that "intense sexual experiences feel really dangerous to me." At that point in the analysis that was as far as he could go in thinking about this experience. I began to understand that his "going through the motions" and his difficulty ejaculating were expressions of both his schizoid defensive system and his sadomasochism. He was terrified of loss of control, of letting someone "into" or letting himself "out of" his closed psychic system. Keeping himself from getting "too excited," a concern he expressed many times in the analysis, helped keep him isolated and therefore safe. He couldn't/wouldn't "let go" with his sexual partners, and he couldn't/wouldn't "let go" with me in the analysis. In the analysis he would always pull back into his schizoid bubble when he got too excited by the good feeling of intimacy with me.

Jack's withholding of his climax, and withholding himself from fully engaging with me, also provided a sadomasochistic pleasure. Both he and his partner (sexual or analytic) suffered from his lack of full engagement. In turn, he suffered from not "getting his needs met" by his partner.

Shortly after his anxiety attack during sex, Jack began to find fault with his girlfriend. She was deficient in so many ways, yet he had to stay with her or he would "crush her soul" because she was in love with him. He was trapped, scared and anxious. I can see now that he displaced his fear of being engulfed by and trapped with me onto this girlfriend. It was her vagina, not mine, that would swallow him up. The analytic relationship began to feel (consciously) safer to him as he acted out his longings, fears and hatreds with his girlfriend.

Because he experienced his girlfriend as the controlling, engulfing Other, I, by contrast, was felt by him to be more benign. He used this splitting to make the analysis a safer place.

The sadomasochistic phase

This sense of safety allowed Jack to be more open with me, expressing his "softness" needs, his need to feel alive and his need to control me. The following is a brief excerpt of a session that occurred the day after his intense, tearful and moving declaration of his need for me to help him.

He says, "Well yesterday really felt good. I mean my depression lifted immediately. I felt alive and completely different. (He elaborates on feeling good). I'm wondering, why you don't do that more. (pause) I wonder why you haven't experimented with me more."

I say, "Experimented with you?"

He says, "Yeah, push me this way or that to see what gets a reaction. Like yesterday you pushed me or, I don't know if it was pushing but I just wondered why you don't experiment more."

I say, "It sounds like you're feeling like I did something to you yesterday."

He says, "Well yeah, what else could it be? What are you thinking?"

I say, "More like something was happening between us."

He says, "Hmm, I'll have to think about that. (pause) But I really think you should push me more. I need to be more stimulated. I don't know why you don't just agree with that. It seems obvious that you should do what you did yesterday more often." He expounded on this theme, getting angrier and more demanding as the session went on.

In effect, the session was under his control. Either I would submit to his demands for me to "do what I did" or I would be purposely depriving him of what he most needed. He rejected every word I offered, every attempt to think with him about yesterday and today. When I tried to reflect back what was happening in the room, he withdrew into a quiet rage until the end of the session.

I could see that the previous day's session was very threatening to Jack. His withdrawal served a variety of functions. It served a regressive function of providing basic protection from engagement with me as a real person, an "objective object". It also helped him re-establish his internal equilibrium by being the controlling, then withholding, Other. I was reminded again of how traumatic contact with the Other felt to him.

As Jack's relationship with his girlfriend came to an end, a new phase of the analysis began. All of his sadistic and masochistic energies poured into the analysis. During this phase I saw more clearly how his schizoid omnipotence and his sadomasochism supported each other. He closed in on himself to a greater degree than I had previously witnessed and experienced. Gone were the sterile days of the "depression report" and the esoteric monologues.

What appeared instead was a level of self-hatred and self-attack that was terrifying for both of us. He mercilessly attacked himself for needing and wanting the girlfriend, for being "deficient" as a man and not able to sustain a relationship. He found proof everywhere he went that he was a "loser" and that no woman would ever want him (that is, no woman that was stimulating enough for him). Every session consisted of his reporting in detail the mental beatings he had given himself since our last session. He described himself to me as feeling severely depressed. He began having suicidal fantasies. He mocked me for offering to help with his pain. He declared that his internal world was the only reality. If I couldn't see that, then I was deluding myself.

And yet, all of this was described to me as a report of what had happened since the previous session. He could not feel it in the room with me. During one of the sessions when we were trying to make sense of this reporting versus feeling it with me in the room he said, "Maybe it would feel too intimate." The next day he reported a dream: He was in a warehouse full of tools and old manufacturing equipment. I was somewhere nearby, maybe in the "main house." As he wandered through the warehouse looking at the equipment he noticed that his pants were gone. He was naked from the waist down. He looked down at his penis and, as he did so, a piece of equipment caught his eye. As he got closer to get a better look, he saw that it was a vise. Inscribed on the top of the vise was the word "HOOD".

His first associative response was a question: "Isn't a hood the name of a part of the vagina or the vulva or something? Isn't it somewhere near the clitoris?" I answered yes. There was a pause, then he said, "I know I was afraid of getting my penis caught in that vise. Or really, that the vise might somehow get hold of my penis. I'm not sure which." As he continued to associate to the dream we were able to talk about his fear of "losing his penis" if he dared feel his horrible feelings with me. That level of intimacy would un-man him. I remembered with him his early fears of giving into "softness," creature comforts, lest they make him feel less masculine. As he put it, he "intellectually understood" why he was afraid of feeling intimate with me, but it remained a theory. He needed to not feel with me. The sado-masochistic solution kept him "hard." It also supported his schizoid system by providing stimulation (painful as it was), thus reducing the need to deal with the outside world. I feared there was no way through this defensive structure.

Jack felt frightened of his suicidal fantasies. They were getting more elaborate. I felt frightened too. Would he really kill himself? As I had done many times before, I reminded him that he could always call me during one of these episodes. He didn't have to go through it alone. His answer was always the same. It would feel emasculating to call me. He would feel like a baby.

The lacerating self-attacks went on month after month. Then one evening I got a message from him. He said he felt like he was losing his mind, that he was terrified of hurting himself, and would I call him back. That evening was the beginning of a new relationship between us. Although it developed in fits and starts, we arrived at a place where he could feel his self-hatred in the room with me. He would cry and writhe on the couch as if in terrible pain as he viciously attacked himself for being a deficient loser, etc. He developed a skin rash over much of his body. He demanded that I put an end to his misery by giving him permission to kill himself. This demand was repeated over and over. He felt that I was cruel to not "sign off" on his suicide so he could finally be free of pain. He tortured himself and he tortured me by not allowing me to "help" by warding me off and insisting on my uselessness to "fix the pain." I sometimes felt like I was sitting with a burn victim in the hospital, horrified at the level of pain I was witnessing. More than ever I had a real sense of his incredible shame for being unable to be loved by his mother. And I got a sense of the incredible rage he felt towards her. As I made interpretations based on these experiences with him, he was able to talk about the pleasure he received when he imagined his parents hearing about his suicide. This revelation opened up a space for us to talk about many of the functions these self-attacks served. He talked about the pleasure of "reveling" in the "orgy" of self-pity and self-hatred. The intensity had an erotic quality to it. It also felt like a warm, familiar blanket that he could wrap himself in. I thought of a quote I read in a book by Novick & Novick (1996) on sadomasochism: "unhappiness smells of home."

We discovered another function of his self-attacks: They warded off the feeling of deadness that he had experienced all of his life. He imagined that if he "gave up" the self-attacks he would have nothing left inside of him. He would be utterly empty. He realized how thrilling it was when he was being the powerful attacker. He was surprised to discover the pleasure he felt when submitting to the attacks. He wondered if he was "addicted" to the self-attacks because of all they provided him. The thought terrified him. There might be no way out but suicide.

I thought of Ogden's reference to Fairbairn and his construct of "addictive love"—the bond between the libidinal ego and the exciting object. As long as Jack continued the self-attacks, he remained in contact with the exciting and withholding internal mother. As Ogden put it, "All of the love and hate that tie these internal objects to one another is entirely the result of the pathological tie of the infant to the unreachable mother who is experienced as not capable of giving or receiving love" (Ogden, 2010, p. 91). Jack's early traumatic experiences with his mother were so very painful. But they were all he had of her. If "unhappiness is the smell of home" then, for Jack, sadomasochism is being with mother.

I realized another function of my samurai beheading fantasy. It allowed me to experience and act out the sadomasochistic (internal) relationship between Jack and his mother. As he used his self-attacks to maintain connection with the internal mother, I managed to maintain a feeling of connection and aliveness with him each time I beheaded him.

Sheer madness

Although the violent self-attacks were unrelenting, they were not unproductive. The erotically tinged penetration by the hard sadistic internal object into the "soft" masochistic internal object produced a monster. And this monster dominated the analysis for many, many months. Although Jack had always scanned his body and face for evidence of unattractiveness, this scanning became an obsession; and, as he did so, he noticed a slight swelling in the jaw area on the left side of his face. He hoped it was cancer because then he could refuse treatment (stay hard) and slowly die while we all (all of us who had harmed him) watched, helpless.

But it wasn't a tumor. His physician said it was a slight muscle buildup most likely caused by clenching his teeth during sleep. He developed a delusion that he was horribly disfigured, disgustingly asymmetrical. The more he obsessed on this (very mild) swelling of the jaw on his face, the larger it seemed to get. His obsession with his face became all-consuming. He spent session after session agonizing about his horrible disfigurement. In some sessions he cried and clutched his face in his hands. In other sessions he lay in bitter silence. He seemed completely lost to the world of reality. I believed that he was experiencing what Balint (1968) describes as the area of the basic fault. His conviction that he was utterly flawed and unlovable dominated his life. He was not able to keep up with the demands of his work, he had trouble sleeping, he had trouble eating. He was re-experiencing his infantile breakdowns, but he would/could not let me help (in the way I wanted to help, that is, through interpretations).

I interpreted his experience of his face as an expression of his self-hatred. I interpreted his experience of his face as re-experiencing his belief that he repulsed his mother and that was why she couldn't love him. I made a lot of interpretations, and each one both enraged him and increased his feeling of futility. He began demanding that I agree with him that he looked like a deformed monster. If I said something like "I see that you feel like a deformed monster," he would become enraged with me. I had to say that he *was* a deformed monster.

I felt completely lost. The pain and rage in the room seemed unbearable. I wanted to make the pain go away for both of us. The critical moment came when Jack sat on the couch, turned, looked at me and said, crying, "Tell me how it looks, tell me, really, how bad it is." Filled with so many emotions, I said, "It's really very mild." His face crumpled in on itself. He lay back down and cried, saying, "It's hopeless, it's really hopeless." At that moment I felt I had failed him completely, though I wasn't sure how. I took his "it's hopeless" comment as confirmation that I had failed him.

I felt horribly guilty for failing him so utterly. I expected him to come to the next session full of rage. Or maybe I hoped he would come to the next session full of rage. But he didn't. He came with a sense of futility that was heart-breaking. For that session and the next he lay silently on the couch. He didn't seem withholding and he didn't seem withdrawn. He seemed actually present, and very, very sad.

We were slowly able to talk about his sense that I had completely let him down. He felt relieved and grateful when I acknowledged what he considered to be my failure, that I had not "seen" him in just the way that his parents had not "seen" him. Haltingly, we began the process of examining my action and his pain.

As we struggled to make sense of and find meaning in what had occurred between us I was able to be more open with Jack when discussing my experience of our interaction. I described the bind I had felt myself to be in, that I understood that he wanted me to see him just the way he saw himself, but I didn't. Over time, as we discussed both his and my experiences, he was able to see the delusional aspect of the experience of his face. He still often felt unattractive, but not deformed. The sense of being a deformed monster came to be an experience that had meaning and could be understood. My previously rejected interpretations concerning his feelings of being profoundly unlovable were reconsidered. He could imagine himself, as a baby, feeling repulsive when his mother withdrew from him during her depressive episodes. The sessions became more alive as he spoke with me instead of at me. More and more often the focus of the sessions concerned his positive and negative feelings about me. More and more often the sessions lived in the here and now. The process was not easy sailing. There were plenty of storms and droughts, loving and hating, fear and gratitude. But these experiences were happening between two live people in the room. It felt that we were sharing an experience of wanting and trying to repair the "damage" we had inflicted on each other. For the most part, the discussions were organized around the way I had failed him by not seeing him exactly the way he wanted me to. However he, too, wanted to make repairs. He expressed his gratitude that I had not given up on him, and that he knew he had been "really mean" sometimes. Over the last year the self-attacks have greatly diminished, though not disappeared; the delusion of disfigurement has become something to look back on and think about. The pain of my not seeing him as he wanted me to see him has become something we refer to as we go through new positive and negative experiences together.

During this fertile period of real contact with Jack I often asked myself why I had felt so strongly that I had failed him, why I felt so guilty about not being able to relieve his pain.

One morning I woke up from a dream about a "bad baby". As I mulled over the dream, realizing that of course I was the "bad baby" in the dream, I asked myself the question: "How was I a bad baby?" At that moment I understood at least some aspects of my reaction to Jack's dream and my sense that I had utterly failed him.

I believe I was in a state of massive identification with him as we entered his area of the basic fault. His unrelenting pain and my inability to relieve it tapped into my area of the basic fault. I had not been able to relieve my parent's depressions, or provide the perfect mirroring they needed to support their fragile self-esteem. My sense of badness for "utterly failing" my parents resurfaced when I could not alleviate Jack's s terrible pain or provide the perfect mirroring he demanded. To my mind, I was failing him. In this parallel process I was also identified with Jack, the "bad baby" who had "utterly failed" to cure his mother's depression.

Of course, it was my very inability to merge with him that produced the positive outcome. The moment he turned to me to ask for "reality" (how bad is it really?) was the critical moment because he was bringing all the weight he could muster to break down the boundary between him and me and pull me into his schizoid/sadomasochistic world. I remained firmly outside the area of his personal omnipotence, and was therefore experienced as an objective object that he could use. My survival of his attempts to break me down facilitated his capacity to bear separateness and external reality.

Recently Jack and I have found ourselves discussing an issue that was paramount when he first began analysis: How can two people be in a relationship without one using/exploiting the other to meet his/her own needs? The content looks to be the same as at the beginning of the analysis, but we both know how different things are now. We are talking together, two people in a room. He said recently, "I was at work the other day and I was thinking about the future, things I want to do, and I realized I had hope. Just like that, I have hope. Life seems pretty good." He continued, "I used to think I would never be able to finish analysis. I imagined quitting it, but not finishing it. I can kind of see the light at the end of the tunnel now, not quitting but finishing." I, too, have begun to see the light at the end of the tunnel. It may be several years away, but I believe in it now in a way I didn't a few years ago.

I am looking forward to continuing this analysis with Jack. I am curious to see what "phases" are ahead of us. And I am happy that Jack and I have faith that we can survive whatever is ahead of us together.

Concluding remarks

My work with this patient has made clear to me the role of sadomasochism in binding and maintaining a closed schizoid psychic system. In addition to this protective function, sadomasochism also reflects and brings alive the trauma of early maternal deprivation. It is through suffering, with the patient, the deadness, the rage, the pain and ultimately the terror of psychic annihilation that allows the patient an experience of "safely not alone". The trauma of contact with the Other can be transformed into an ability for genuine contact with external reality. Woody Allen once quipped, "I hate reality, but it's the only place I can get a good steak dinner." For my patient, reality became a place where he could make genuine contact with the Other and finally get his needs met.

References

Balint, M. (1968). *The Basic Fault.* Evanston, IL: Northwestern University Press.

Eigen, M. (2004). *The Electrified Tightrope.* London: Karnac.

Fairbairn, W.R.D. (1944). Endopsychic structure considered in terms of object relationships. *International Journal of Psychoanalysis,* 27: 70–93.

Fairbairn, W.R.D. (1952). *Psychoanalytic Studies of the Personality.* London & New York: Routledge.

Freud, S. (1915). Instincts and their vicissitudes. *Standard Edition 14*: 143.

Novick, J. & Novick, K. (1996). *Fearful Symmetry.* Northvale, NJ: Jason Aronson.

Odgen, T.H. (2010). Why read Fairbairn? *International Journal of Psychoanalysis,* 91: 101–118.

Reik, A. (1941). *Masochism in Modern Man.* New York: Farrar & Rinehart.

Sartre, J.-P. (1957). *Being and Nothingness.* New York: Philosophical Library.

Winnicott, D.W. (1971). *Playing and Reality.* London & New York: Routledge.

Yalom, I. (1980). *Existential Psychotherapy.* New York: Basic Books.

Chapter 3

Stubborn love

Lori O'Brien

Introduction

Trauma occurs when the ego is totally unprepared for a traumatizing event of an external kind. The stimulus barrier is broken, and the ego is overwhelmed with a degree of anxiety that it is unable to master. When a very young child is threatened by a degree of pervasive anxiety with which he is unable to deal, and which can only be assuaged by the ministrations of a mother who detects the source of that anxiety, there is a prototype for later fears of annihilation (Yorke, 1986). This experience creates a flood of excitation, both physiologically and intrapsychically. In a perverse sense, this vegetative excitation may be confused in later life with erotic longing and sexual arousal. The vegetative aspect relates not to a thinking mind, but rather to an infantile state of physiological and proprioceptive experiences. It is in this manner that a sexual connection with a replicate of the original traumatizing bad object enlivens and reduces the terror of disintegration in adulthood.

In this chapter, I will describe a brief overview of the theoretical understanding of early psychological trauma and its aftermath. I will present case examples of two patients who suffered pre- and postnatal developmental trauma. In both cases, the effects of early traumatic experiences intensified the patients' compulsion to seek love objects similar to those of inadequate caretakers, and to attach themselves to situations which replicate the insufficient environmental nurturing previously experienced. In both cases, there has been a stubborn insistence that this particular form of love object is the only option. There remains a predominant delusion, that this love object can be controlled, manipulated and modified into a more loving, protective and nourishing caretaker. Existing relationships represent a tie between self and fantasy, rather than self and other.

Winnicott (1971) described the concept of a transitional object, to be considered both part of the self and not part of the self. If traumatic experiences in the environment prevent the baby from relinquishing the sense of the object as part of the self, a connection to reality outside of the self is limited. The patients I will describe struggle to possess their tenuous objects as part of the self and, therefore, are not able to use them as developmental tools toward building a sense of autonomy and an awareness of reality.

I will conclude with notes on the treatment implications suggested by my work with these patients. From the beginning, forming a therapeutic alliance with each of them was threatened by my inability to enliven, or excite, in a familiar manner. I felt "too available". My interest in them felt intrusive. My ability to listen appeared persecutory. Additionally, the analytic frame felt unyielding. Any attempt to maintain consistent boundaries would trigger overwhelming anxiety, and fear of dependence. It was important that I create what Bollas (1987) termed an intermediate space, where there was a sense of me "as of" the self, yet other. In this way, I might be used as a true, transitional object where the waters of reality might be tested.

Infantile trauma: repetitive and pervasive

The question of early trauma, and its effects on maturation and development, is a large and complex one. Childhood trauma involves some form of threatened or actual injury to the mind or body, the loss of an important person, the withdrawal of their needed love or the threat of self-punishment (Portuges & Hollander, 2011).

Recent psychobiological and neurological studies indicate that infantile trauma may begin as early as life itself, in the womb. According to Schore (2000), prenatal maltreatment or neglect compromises cognitive and emotional development of the infant. The maturation of the infant's brain is experience dependent, and is embedded in the attachment relationship from the beginning. The pregnant mother acts as an external, psychobiological regulator of the growth of the infant's development. Further, prenatal experiences are likely to have a lifelong impact when they are followed by reinforcing conditions or interactional trauma.

Piontelli (1992) conducted ultrasound studies which support a continuum between pre- and postnatal life. Meltzer & Williams (1988) claim that both physical and emotional experiences in infancy are registered in the mind, "like shales in a piece of timber mark early periods of drought," and can be represented symbolically in dream thought. Recent studies have focused on the dream life of neonates, suggesting an unconscious registration of experiences occurring in the womb (Morgan, 1995). Wilfred Bion suggested that fetal memories suffer the "fate of anonymity" (Grotstein, 2007). Symptoms originate in the prenatal self and erupt in the postnatal self.

Although prenatal neurobiological trauma is beyond the scope of this chapter, it is often the natural precursor to the attachment and relational trauma later seen in the treatment room of psychoanalysts. For patients who have experienced prenatal and/or early infantile trauma, there is often no language for what has been experienced. A bad object/environment is better than no environment at all. Further, the resulting threat of disintegration, death and meaninglessness strengthens the tie to the toxic environment. Freud (1914) articulated the unconscious compulsion to repeat in action that which cannot be remembered. The repetition compulsion is both a defense against remembering and an opportunity to recreate the traumatic experience in an effort to gain control of it, or modify it, to a more positive outcome.

Mitchell (1988) suggested a specific compulsion to recreate as closely as possible the dynamics of the relationship with the bad object. Those suffering from prenatal or infantile trauma may seek to recreate pathological environments as a defense against a sense of deadness. Fairbairn (1943) stated that, for the helpless infant, a bad object is better than no object, and may be the only thing standing between the infant and abject terror or death.

Vicissitudes of cumulative trauma in interpersonal relations

> Without object relations, the ego itself cannot develop.
>
> (Guntrip, 1969, p. 20)

Khan (1974) postulated that repetitive trauma in the early mother–child relationship forms a dynamic substratum in developing particular character pathologies. He saw the mother as a protective shield, and claimed that her inability to protect the child from a particular incidence of stress is insignificant in and of itself, but that cumulative impingements distort ego development and assault the infant's psyche-soma in a way the infant has no means of protecting itself from.

Analysts working with patients repeating traumatic relationships experienced in early childhood are only too aware of the stubborn reverence the patient exhibits toward his/her toxic environment. To address the reality of abuse, cruelty or demeaning experiences is to confront the patient with a reality too harsh to bear. The lack of ego strength and inability to tolerate disillusionment prevent the patient from accepting the analyst's interpretations.

Balint (1937) stressed that the aim of all human striving is to find harmony with the environment. If the environment is toxic, how then does one find harmony? Cumulative trauma is experienced and stored as memories, which are dissociated if overwhelming to the fragile and developing ego. Grotstein (2007) claimed that prenatal memories are inaccessible to the conscious mind. Massive repression is employed to maintain the prenatal amnesia of traumatic stimuli and find homeostasis and harmony.

To accept the other as a separate being, out of one's control, is terrifying. The other's badness is disavowed, and fantasies of love, nurturing and protection replace reality. There is an insistent belief that the object is part of the self. The relationship is not one with another person, but rather with a fantasy of that person. Stark (2015) claims that it is rage at the other's separateness that fuels the relentlessness with which the object is pursued. The traumatized individual is not only enacting a masochistic repetition of dependence on an unavailable caretaker, but is also fueled by sadistic urges to control and remake the caretaker over into the needed and desired loving object. Stark describes a relentless hope that maybe, this time, the response will be the desired one that, maybe this time, the object will provide.

Two case studies

Case one: Michael

The case of Michael will illustrate the pattern of tenacious attempts to rewrite a traumatic early history through a series of relationships chosen in order to finally control and possess the elusive love object and remake it into a nurturing, caring and available one. Unfortunately, Michael is unable to experience his partners as separate beings, with their own needs, desires and drives, and is unable to avoid the calamitous results, time after time.

Michael was referred to me by a medical doctor who had been treating him for headaches and irritable bowel syndrome for some years. The doctor was frustrated with Michael because he refused medication for anxiety and depression. The doctor felt Michael's psychological symptoms were exacerbating his physical symptoms. Michael eventually called me after a difficult break up with his girlfriend of five years. He told me his heart was broken, he could not function and he did not think he could bring himself to speak about it. He was convinced that, if he spoke of his grief, he would fall into such a state that he would not be able to go on.

Michael, a 32-year-old successful money manager, came from a background laced with early trauma. He was the eldest of three, with two younger sisters, raised on the East Coast. His father was a narcissistic real estate developer, and his mother had been a successful fashion model. Michael learned that during her pregnancy with him, his mother had smoked pot and drank alcohol heavily. He heard from his grandmother that he had almost died in the womb. He had been entwined in the umbilical cord. He also learned that his mother had two miscarriages prior to marrying his father, and had been depressed and unsure about having more children.

Michael was born prematurely, and spent two weeks in a neonatal intensive care unit (NICU), in an incubator. His mother suffered postpartum depression and was unable to visit or hold him during his early months. Michael has no recollection of who might have cared for him. After Michael was brought home from the hospital, he felt his mother had no interest in him and blamed him for the onset of her depression. He said, "I was left alone most of the time. I'm a thinker. I've always had to figure things out for myself."

Michael lived in a mind full of fantasies, which allowed him to put a positive spin on the situation. However, he had never thought about how he had internalized early, overwhelming anxieties, and what effect they wreaked on his body. He invested enormous amounts of energy into maintaining his "positive" outlook. Michael repressed his grief and rage at a mother who could not nurture or protect him.

When Michael was one and a half his mother had a brief affair, and left the home for around six months. Michael thinks his grandmother came to stay with him so that his father, a high-stress workaholic, would not feel interfered with. He reports this as "no big deal" because, somewhere inside, he knew his mother loved him and would return. She returned, and had an intense, renewed love affair with his father, who took her on numerous trips to Europe, the Bahamas and Tahiti over the course of the next few years. During this time, his mother became pregnant twice, with his two sisters, and his sisters became the products of his parents "real" marriage, after his parents were "sure" about each other. Michael describes his mother as gorgeous, the life of the party, adventurous and free spirited. He told me that she is most attached to his middle sister, Annette, who is just like her. Annette, a burgeoning model herself, often smoked pot with their mother.

Michael came to his first session on time, immaculately dressed and impeccably groomed. He was handsome and extremely stylish. However, he appeared somewhat shy and dejected. He related that he felt hopeless, and was having difficulty breathing as he spoke. I felt anxious and unsure if I would have the capacity to contain all that was being presented. I immediately sensed that these were the feelings of a new mother, faced with a disorganized and fragile infant.

Over the course of the next few weeks, Michael reported to me that he had been in love three times. He thought of each of these women as his soul mate, and he only felt truly alive when he was with them. The first relationship lasted eight years, and ended when his girlfriend, who had repeatedly cheated on him, finally left him for another man. His second relationship was an intensely passionate affair with a woman who sounded sociopathic. She stole money out of his wallet, borrowed art from his house which she sold for cash, and was arrested for credit card fraud, which he helped her to "pay restitution" for so she would not get in trouble. I wanted to interpret that he was repeatedly "paying restitution" for his mother so that he could maintain the idealized fantasies he had of her; yet I sensed that Michael's idealization was holding him together in some way.

This girlfriend also flirted shamelessly in front of him, including kissing other men. She wanted him to be turned on by it, but he said it put him in a deep depression. He tried hard to impress her, and even bought her a car so that she would see him as more valuable than other men; but he eventually broke up with her after she shamed him miserably in front of his colleagues by performing a pseudo lap dance on his assistant at a party. Michael remains heartbroken that he could not figure out how to make this relationship work. Sex with her made him feel alive. He still ruminates about what he could have done differently.

As Stark (2015) proposed, it is not only masochism which fuels the ongoing attempts to keep the dysfunctional relationship alive, but also the relentless hope that maybe this time, with this effort and this extreme measure, the love object will respond differently. Michael had witnessed his mother flirt and drink with other men, which he equated to her abandonment of him. This time, Michael was not a helpless child but, rather, a successful businessman who could woo his lover with extravagant gifts. He held fast to the fantasy that he would be able to "wow" his love object, and that his reward would be her devotion and affection.

His most recent relationship lasted for three years. She was a charismatic artist he met at an art opening, and he fell in love "at first sight". He did not ask for her number right away, but kept abreast of her art shows and her whereabouts on the internet. He fantasized about being with her, and had a vivid dream of them lying on the floor, her on top of him stroking his hair, saying she "would always take care of him". She cooked for him, and encouraged him to smoke pot. I thought of the mother who smoked pot when pregnant with Michael, and of how he envied his mother and sister Annette enjoying each other while smoking. I was keenly aware that the power of this relationship dynamic had washed over Michael with a blissful haze, brought on by much more than the simple effects of cannabis. In the throes of love with this woman, he felt loved. He said, "I was in a state of bliss and happiness."

He recognized that he immediately sensed feeling possessive and jealous. He said:

> I know it's horrible, but I wanted to lock her away all to myself. I rented her an art studio, but got angry when she invited other guys over. I threw her an art show, and then got mad when she invited some of her exes. She was always telling me I was insecure. I kept trying not to be, but I could not help it. We fought constantly, and my stomach issues got worse. I ended up in the hospital with numerous tests to see if I had colon cancer. She only came to visit me for ten minutes. Friends and family told me to lose her. I got out of the hospital and wanted to reignite our loving feelings. A client of hers offered to open a retail space for her to showcase her art. She began to show him much attention. It was making me emotionally and physically ill. I was desperate, and bought her a big rock. I asked her to marry me. She smiled and said how sweet. I didn't get an answer. The next night, I followed her. Can you believe this shit? Me. Following my girlfriend in a rental car. I found out everything I suspected was true. She went to this guy's house and stayed overnight. I went home and cried for three days. I got really drunk and called her, and she said, "let's talk tomorrow because you're really tipsy." I think I just wanted her to see how desperately in love with her I was. I still want to figure out a way to make it work. I still see us getting back together.

I interpreted that there was an earlier relationship he was trying to fix. It occurred to me that, much like Stark had proposed, Michael was fueled by an unconscious rage that this woman was incapable of loving him the way he wanted, the way he wanted his mother to love and appreciate him. His repeated attempts to "win her over" were negating the real her, the separate her who would do what she wished, with whom she wished, no matter what Michael was willing to do.

Michael's traumatic history suggests that his rejection and abandonment provided ample opportunity to fuel primitive fantasies of an internal, loving mother, under his control and subject to his whims. His traumatic loss occurred so early that it was unimaginable to his developing mind. Michael repeated frantically in his adulthood his situation with a toxic and unavailable mother in order to coerce her into attending to his needs. Kernberg (1995) suggests that the remarkable absence of any loving, concerned, parental object leads to primitive fantasies of power as the only assurance of an alternative to total submission and helplessness in the face of a sadistic object. Here was an extraordinarily attractive and successful man who had many choices in his romantic life. However, the "right one" was inevitably the seductive and narcissistic vixen, who both "brought him to life" and then abandoned him.

As Piontelli (1992) suggested from her prenatal observations, when a baby experiences trauma in the womb, as Michael did, repetitive behavioral characteristics are set from the start. Michael was surrounded by a toxic amniotic fluid, his mother suffering mood swings and alcohol dependence. His first sensory object, the umbilical cord, on which he depended to survive, was wound around him in a near lethal manner. The earliest trauma replays itself over and over in Michael's life, where he clings to the most toxic form of connections.

The accumulation of intrauterine trauma, the absence of a maternal object during incubation and the abandonment by his mother in early childhood left Michael with no option but to create a fantasy world to contain his infantile terrors. In this world, Michael's fantasy mother would return because, wherever she was and no matter what she was doing, she was loving him.

The dream Michael related after meeting his last love was that he was having his hair stroked, and hearing soothing, protective words. These powerful words were attached in fantasy to the new love object. She was imbued with all the qualities of Michael's fantasy lover/mother, and to wake Michael from this dream, as friends and family members had attempted, was to shatter the fantasy that sustained Michael through a terrifying early life. To wake would be to face the reality of the limited and separate other, who did not exist to soothe and comfort him, but rather to pursue her own separate interests.

Winnicott (1989) claimed that, in anticipation of loss, we see an exaggerated use of a transitional object, as a denial of the threat of becoming meaningless. Transitional objects gradually become decathected in normal development, as outside interests evolve; but for Michael the threat of disintegration fueled his grasp on them.

Michael was deeply concerned about who came into the consulting room after him. He often lingered to use the restroom so he could see who followed him. I interpreted that he was concerned about the siblings who followed, as they were the siblings born of "real love" from the "real marriage". They were the children I was prepared for, and would take seriously. His struggle against feelings of rejection were understandable given the horrible reality of his early dependency.

Although Michael dreams of a soothing, nurturing love which will ameliorate his internal terror, nothing will erase the wounds of his past. However, if I am a good enough mother/analyst, I may be able to create a space filled not with toxins and treachery, but with understanding and reliability, so that if Michael is able to wake from the "dream he lives in" there will be a good enough mother to "hold him" as he grieves and experiences the real disappointments from his past.

Case 2: Guinnevere

Guinnevere was referred to me by a couples' therapist she had seen briefly at the request of her partner. She was in her early 20s, with full body tattoos, multiple piercings and long dark hair, which she purposely left unwashed. She was named after the Crosby, Stills and Nash song "Guinnevere", who had green eyes, and was wild and free. Guinnevere sarcastically stated that her "hippie" parents had imagined her as a wild bird, free to fly without limits. She said "translation—we don't want to be burdened by a pain in the ass baby. The reality was, I think I just kept falling out of the nest."

Guinnevere had a series of brief, intensely sexual affairs, with both men and women, which ended "painfully and dramatically." She wanted help understanding why, after her last relationship ended, she began having dreams and fantasies of having been sexually abused. She had made three suicidal gestures in her teens, two with drug overdoses and a third by cutting the veins in both of her wrists and getting in the bath. She watched herself bleed for a moment, then called a roommate and asked her to get help. She was taken to the Emergency Room, and described the paramedics as irritated, rather than caring toward her. Her hunger for a maternal object, capable of responding to her desperate state of near death, was evident when she related this sad event.

In our initial phone conversation, when discussing potential times to meet, she selected one of the times I offered and replied, "Sounds good, whatever, man." This phrase "whatever, man" was used in response to almost all of my interpretations, and symbolized her capitulation to others' whims, and as a mask to conceal her anger and aggression, particularly toward men.

Guinnevere was raised by parents who were in and out of rehab during her infancy and childhood. They never married or were monogamous, but remain good friends. She was born at home, with a midwife, and her mother used self-prescribed narcotics in lieu of an epidural. As an infant, neighbors twice rushed Guinnevere to the hospital due to finding her in a deep sleep, possibly unconscious. There was no maternal or paternal caretaker to respond to her fragile state. As a child, she slept for many long hours, "as if she had taken halcyon." As an adult, she has the belief that she needs 12 hours of sleep a night in order to function. She said to me, "I love sleep. It's my favorite hobby." It is unclear what specific drugs Guinnevere was exposed to in the womb; however, she herself has struggled with addiction to cocaine and alcohol for the majority of her young adult life, but is currently sober.

According to Auhagen-Stephanos (2013), prenatal experience is stored in the body's memory, and may unconsciously be repeated. Guinnevere's intrauterine experience suggests not only a physiological predisposition to addiction, but also an emotional craving in body memory of numbing the pain and terror she experienced at separation. Her fragile connection to her life instinct was repeatedly bombarded by an ambivalent "whatever, man" attitude toward life and death, and replays itself over and over in her laissez-faire mode of self-care, presentation and suicidal gestures.

Guinnevere's mother played several musical instruments quite well, and took frequent road trips with groups she played in. At those times, Guinnevere was either left with her father and his other girlfriends or stayed with her paternal grandmother. In her recent couples' therapy, Guinnevere began having dreams that her father's girlfriends asked her to participate in an orgy with them, while her father watched, and that her father received fellatio in the shower while she sat on the bathroom floor. She felt that these were not true events; but they disturbed her, and she wanted me to help her figure out why she was having them.

Guinnevere describes her relationship history as "a hot mess" of events. Her longest relationship was with a boyfriend in high school, who was working at a Jamba Juice store with her. The relationship lasted three months, but he stole her car keys one night while she was passed out, and got in an accident, totaling her car. He broke it off with her so that he would not have to pay her back.

Guinnevere describes men as either wolves or dogs. Wolves are wild and independent. Dogs like her too much, and follow her around. She is only attracted to the wolves. Her few, brief sexual encounters with women were sweet, but boring and unsatisfying. In the transference, Guinnevere experiences me also as boring and unsatisfying. In the transference, I was not the aggressive, exciting wolf that enlivens and excites her. My therapeutic nest had constraining guard rails, and while she wouldn't fall out, she feared she wouldn't fly.

Guinnevere described an older woman with whom she had a one-night stand. She stated firmly, "Don't tell me I'm looking for a mother substitute. One mother was plenty for me." When I asked her why she thought I would tell her that, she replied, "Cause it's in all the psycho literature man, but I don't buy into that shit." She told me she was reading up on psychology because she did not want me to have anything "over on her." When I asked her to expand upon how having one mother was enough for her, she related that "It was too much work." She always had to be the adult.

> My mother was the original "hot mess," but kinda fragile you know. Guys were always taking advantage of her, so I kept tabs on her, worried that she'd be high and some asshole guy would rape her. My dad was too much of a loser to look after her.

Guinnevere's fears of dependency were grounded in the harsh reality that there had been no one to "look after her" when she was "kinda fragile." It took many years for me to be able to interpret this dynamic back to her. She identified with her mother in her dreams of sexual abuse.

Guinnevere's urgent hunger and unmet oral needs were often projected onto others chosen, and found sexually enticing, specifically based on their neediness of her. She felt safer when the sexual other was the dependent party in the relationship. Her flight from sexual partners who had been "conquered" may have also been an attempt to protect and preserve them from her oral greed. She split off her aggression onto predatory "wolves".

According to Kernberg (1995), there is an intensification of erotic longing when there has been an early experience of unrequited love. In Guinnevere's case, this continuum of brief, sexually intense relationships exemplifies her overwhelming, early longings. It is clear that Guinnevere was exposed to numerous precocious sexual encounters, and experienced the act of intercourse as dominated by male aggression. Her dreams suggested an Oedipal wish to participate as a voyeur outside of herself who witnessed things which were "unseeable" and "unspeakable" to her preverbal, and helpless, self. Freud (1915) claimed that patients who experienced early trauma, and had withdrawn their libidinal cathexis into their own ego, exhibit narcissistic personalities and are resistant to dependency in the transference. For patients who have been sexually abused, any sexualized, or other, longings for the analyst may be experienced as humiliating and shameful.

Wurmser (1994) described the genetic triad of shame in which weakness, dirtiness and defectiveness are the core experiences. Guinnevere identified herself in this way. She kept herself unwashed and unkempt, to exhibit her underlying feelings of dirtiness. She described her sexual self as "dirty" and "disgusting." She tried to cover up her feelings of defectiveness by acting superior and parental. In the transference, she experienced me as being appalled or disgusted with her. As Lewis (1971) claimed, feelings of shame can lead to rage when one has been abandoned or excluded. In fantasy, Guinnevere attempts to convert her powerlessness and humiliation into a pseudo-strength with her "whatever, man" attitude.

In treatment, as tenuous as our connection was at times, Guinnevere was able to use my consistency to eventually feel that I was an object she could use and reuse in the manner of a transitional object. She was able to cancel, arrive late, insult and rage at me in envious attacks. She cried, sat silent and acted as if she didn't care. The boundaries of the therapeutic frame served to form a space where we could begin to explore how Guinnevere's pseudo-confidence was a mask for the helplessness and vulnerability she felt. Grounded in the history of her suicidal gestures was the fear that she might not be able to maintain her tenuous tie to reality, or to life itself. There was an ambivalent wish that she might one day stay "asleep" forever. To open her eyes to the reality of her fragility and undeveloped self—pushed out of the nest, into a world of wolves—was too terrifying to face.

After eight years of work, Guinnevere has begun to experience me as a separate entity. She recently remarked that she noticed another patient of mine entering. She wondered how she had never noticed that before. She said, "Like duh, you see other patients." She felt that perhaps she would not have been able to stand it before. She wanted to think of "us" as just "us", in a bubble. We were able to use this experience as a symbol of all the random women that "pulled up" to her home to have sex with her father, and how intolerable this must have felt. She realized how scared she was to know that I had other "little girls", ones that may not be as dirty and defective as she was. She worried that "these girls" would seduce my attentions away from her.

Recently Guinnevere came to session with her guitar to sing me a song. She sang about being rudely awakened from a dream into a world she found horrifying. She smiled, and said I ruined her life because I brought her "awake" to how "fucked up" her childhood was. She felt everything was easier when she was "asleep", and began to articulate in words her ambivalence about "getting better" and "growing up". She said, "Being sober is hard. I have to feel all this anger and pain. There are days I wish I could just go back to sleep."

Guinnevere has fallen off the wagon a few times, but for the most part is able to work hard on her sobriety. She has formed a more positive identification with the good parts of her parents, their creativity and musical talent. She is tutoring underprivileged kids in guitar, and is doing some of her own song writing. She is working hard to imagine how she might find someone she doesn't have to "fix". She says sometimes, she is so mad at me for opening her eyes to things because she may never be able to "get laid" again, but that therapy and AA have also probably saved her life, which might be worth saving.

Transference, countertransference and treatment implications

> The development of the socially higher forms of love derive as a consequence of adaptation to reality.
>
> (Balint, 1949, p. 257)

In working with patients from traumatic backgrounds, one may note that the initial interest in forming a therapeutic alliance is when the illusion of oneness with their love object has broken, and the eternal optimism of transforming the "other" into a desperately needed caretaker has faltered. Both of the patients I describe had a series of relationships repeating previous trauma. They had failed to modify the familiar love object into a loving and protective caretaker. The "good mother" of their earlier infantile fantasies did not emerge. After repeated futile attempts, the losses piled up, and re-traumatized old wounds, until there was a desperate measure taken to try something different—therapy.

Balint (1949) claims that in the earliest forms of love the object is recognized, but not its self-interests. Only after a gradual development of a reality sense is there a gradual development of true object love. Bollas (1987) suggests that the growth of a sense of reality, of "internal" and "external" and of self and object, provides for psychic continuity. If this continuity is achieved, then the task of the good enough environment/mother (or analyst substitute) is achieved. Bollas refers to the analyst/mother as the transformational mother. She is not a "thing" out there, but rather an agent of change or transformation. In order to achieve this, the therapeutic stance requires a flexible, yet consistent frame. The patient must feel he/she has enough control to tolerate the feelings of helplessness and dependency which inevitably arise.

In *The Basic Fault*, Balint (1968) stressed that the preconditions for a patient's successful internalization of interpretations is a fairly good ego structure. For those patients who have experienced preverbal trauma, the ego remains fragile, and the patient is unable to experience verbal interpretations in a useful manner. He suggested that the patient be allowed to regress to states of primary love, where the boundaries between the mother and baby are blurred, and fantasies of oneness abound. Here, the analyst fosters anew a more harmonious sense of oneness, which may stimulate a willingness of the patient to accept reality. This willingness must arise from a non-toxic environment, co-created by the patient and the analyst. The analyst must be able to provide a flexible, consistent and contained environment in order for the patient to develop. For patients traumatized preverbally, care must be taken with interpretations. Rushing in to verbalize early traumatic, proprioceptive experiences may re-traumatize the patient, regardless of the sensitivity offered to provide them in an empathic manner.

Khan (1973) reinforced this premise in suggesting the role of illusion in the analytic space for patients who cannot use language. My own experience with these patients suggests that allowing the patient to transfer the idealized, and the most denigrated parts of the self, and the internalized mother is the key element in understanding and transforming the early traumatic experiences. An accumulation of traumatic experiences creates resistance to growth. The transformation from fantasy to accepting reality, and the capacity to experience others as separate beings, requires the analyst's capacity to contain and wait. The patient may require a great deal of time to develop the capacity to grieve, and to tolerate the disillusionment inherent in real connections with other human beings.

Conclusion

> Analysis is not just a simple understanding of one feeling or one reaction or one trauma, but really to understand the total existence of the other.
>
> (Bolgar in Diamond, 2011, p. 291)

Life does not appear to spare any of us the experience of trauma; but for those who suffer impingements in their prenatal or early infantile life the effects are particularly destructive. If one has not achieved sufficient ego strength to navigate the inevitable pains and losses to come, there is an incapacity to form healthy connections, and a persistent pattern of repetitive losses and disappointments. From the primitive experience of the fetus, whose earliest connection to life is the intrauterine environment, to the ministrations, or lack thereof, of early caretakers an infant is dependent on his/her early environment for physiological and psychological survival.

Psychoanalysis offers an opportunity to transform the rigid and repetitive defense system, set early on in the service of survival. The analyst's healthy respect for the primitive defenses, which may have been the patient's only hope to live, and the consistent, reliable and organized frame provide a new opportunity for connection. If we are willing to "be" in the co-created space, with our traumatized patients, we may be able to help them to move toward symbolizing, in words, the preverbal terrors previously experienced and repressed. In this manner, patients may find freedom from the prison of internal fantasies created to sustain them in their earliest life.

References

Auhagen-Stephanos, U. (2013). Inside the mother's womb: The mother-embryo dialogue. *The Female Body: Inside and Outside*, I. Moeslein-Teising & F.T. Salo (eds.). London: Karnac, 153–167.

Balint, A. (1949). Love for the mother and mother-love. *International Journal of Psychoanalysis*. 30: 251–259.

Balint, M. (1937). Early developmental states of the ego, primary object of love. *Primary Love and Psycho-Analytic Technique*. London: Tavistock.

Balint, M. (1968). *The Basic Fault: Therapeutic Aspects of Regression.* New York: Brunner/Mazel.
Bollas, C. (1987). *The Shadow of the Object: Psychoanalysis of the Unthought Known.* New York: Columbia University Press.
Diamond, M. (2011). A centenarian's retrospective on psychoanalysis: An interview with Hedda Bolgar. *The Second Century of Psychoanalysis: Evolving Perspectives on Therapeutic Action*, M.J. Diamond, & C. Christian (eds.). London: Karnac, 279–305.
Fairbairn, W.R.D. (1943). The repression and the return of bad objects. *Psychoanalytic Studies of the Personality.* London: Tavistock, 1952.
Freud, S. (1914). Remembering, repeating and working through. *Standard Edition 12*: 145–156. London: Hogarth Press.
Freud, S. (1915). Repression. *Standard Edition 14*: 73–104. London: Hogarth Press.
Guntrip, H.J.S. (1969). *Schizoid Phenomena, Object-Relations and the Self.* New York: International Universities Press.
Grotstein, J. (2007). *A Beam of Intense Darkness.* London: Karnac.
Kernberg, O. (1995). *Love Relations.* New Haven, CT: Yale University Press.
Khan, M. (1974). *The Privacy of Self.* London: Hogarth Press.
Khan, M. (1973). The role of illusion in the analytic space and process. *Annual of Psychoanalysis, Vol. 1.* New York: Quadrangle, 231–246.
Lewis, H. (1971). *Shame and Guilt in Neurosis.* New York: International Universities Press.
Meltzer, D. & Williams, M.H. (1988). *The Apprehension of Beauty.* Old Ballechine, Strathtay: Clunie Press.
Mitchell, S. (1988). *Relational Concepts in Psychoanalysis: An Integration.* Cambridge, MA: Harvard University Press.
Morgan, C.W. (1995). Dreams in the fetus and the newborn. Paper presented at LAISPS. Los Angeles, California.
Piontelli, A. (1992). *From Fetus to Child: An Observational and Psychoanalytic Study.* London: Routledge.
Portuges, S. & Hollander, N. (2011). The therapeutic action of resistance in analysis: Interpersonalizing and socializing Paul Gray's close process attention technique. *The Second Century of Psyschoanalysis: Evolving Perspectives on Therapeutic Action*, M.J. Diamond & C. Christian (eds.). London: Karnac, 71–95.
Schore, A.N. (2000). The effects of early relational trauma on right brain development, affect regulation and infant mental health. *Infant Mental Health Journal*, 22: 201–269.
Stark, M. (2015). *Acceptance, Forgiveness and the Capacity to Relent.* International Psychotherapy Institute.
Winnicott, D.W. (1971). *Playing and Reality.* London: Tavistock.
Winnicott, D.W. (1989). *Psycho-Analytic Explorations.* Cambridge, MA: Harvard University Press.
Wurmser, L. (1994). *The Mask of Shame.* New York: Jason Aronson.
Yorke, C. (1986). Reflections on the problem of psychic trauma. *Psychoanalytic Study of the Child*, 41: 221–236.

Chapter 4

Finding the impulse: healing from infantile trauma

Judy K. Eekhoff

Patients who have been traumatized as infants present in the consulting room as difficult to reach. Depending upon the stage of their recovery, they appear passive, overly compliant and eager to please. They seem to find their initiative in others, taking their cues from the environment and not feeling their own healthy impulses. The desire to connect with others or the ability to connect with themselves seems to be stunted. As they heal in their therapy, impulses return and they must learn, much as young children do, to manage the turmoil these impulses stimulate. These are the moments in the treatment during which impasses occur, for coming alive is terrifying and enraging. Coming alive is overwhelming and traumatizes the patient again.

This chapter uses a clinical example to demonstrate the process of recovering lost impulses from infancy and dealing with the overwhelming affect that is evoked in psychoanalytic treatment. Ordinary mothers of newborns pay attention to their infant's every gesture. They notice contact. They interpret lip movements, head turns, breaths and sounds. They know there is meaning in their newborn's impulses, and they look for that meaning. When they cannot find it, they seek it, touching a cheek with a nipple, caressing a head with a hand, looking into baby's eyes and cooing. They call a baby forth, saying, "Come out, Baby." When an infant cries, a mother quickly learns what each cry means and attends. And when an infant cries, he is calling forth his mother, saying, as only an infant can, "Are you my mother?", "Come, mommy, come." Adults who were separated at birth from their mothers have within their internal worlds an infant that was not called forth or met, an absent or indifferent mother, and a raging inferno of unmediated and undifferentiated affect. Most of them do not know this, but their partners, if they have partnered, do. If they come to therapy, they may say "something is missing." Although they may be bright and engaging in a superficial sense, they may complain of not reaching their potential or of being passive in their endeavors. Analysts who attempt to reach these patients do so by working in the moment, in relationship to the coming and going contact as well as transference and countertransference between them. Analysts who work with the infant in these adults must answer the infantile call for a lost mother and become the mother who calls them forth from the silent depths of themselves. To become the lost mother of infancy, the analyst must use her intuition and her imagination, which are informed by contact with the patient and by the countertransference.

According to Bion (1962), the boundary between self and other, between self and self, between conscious and unconscious is maintained by the contact barrier. The contact barrier is itself formed from making meaning of sensate experience, what Bion calls alpha working on beta. The contact barrier is permeable and fluid. It is constantly shifting, just as our states of mind and our vertices are constantly changing. Our contact barrier protects us from a sensory world fraught with danger where we are constantly being impinged upon by internal and external physical and psychic reality. The combination of somatic and mental experience without a good enough contact barrier over-stimulates and overwhelms us. Our alpha functioning develops in relationship with an external other, beginning in the first moments of sentience within the mother's body. At birth, our alpha function continues to develop with contact or in relationship to the perception or awareness of our senses as well as through the engagement of our parents, most specifically our mothers. When alpha function is sufficient to continually maintain a good enough contact barrier, containment makes learning possible. Bion developed his model of container and contained using the mother's containing function of the infant's sensory experience as a representation of the process. Learning to dream or to play with our sensory world in relationship develops our alpha function. Alpha function, which enables us to play with language and use our imaginations, is what makes us uniquely human. Alpha function is much more than thinking. It is reverie that informs thinking. It is much more than dreaming, although dreaming is a factor.

When our alpha functioning becomes compromised, we are confused. We defend against the confusion by retreating to the world of the senses where we are aware of everything without finding meaning in it. Our awareness is not the same as consciousness, for awareness can threaten us with losing our relationship with ourselves as well as with others. Consciousness is about having a relationship with our selves as well as with others. Unmediated awareness of our perceptions overwhelms our minds and forces us to defend via concrete thinking, where our world becomes rigid and tight, limited by what we cannot tolerate. Patients who have been prematurely separated from their mothers at birth and left too long alone with their somatic experience become attached via hyper-vigilance to the sights, sounds and sensations around them. Their awareness impedes their development of consciousness. They also may become attached to their own thoughts in what Esther Bick (1968) calls the second skin phenomenon. As I have said (Eekhoff, 2019, p. 80):

> I believe, with Klein and Bion, that the infant is born object related and with a very primitive capacity for representation. I believe that the infant

> is born with a primitive capacity for binding affects. Binding holds the affective charges together, mediating their intensity (Freud, 1920). This suggests to me that the infant is born with an embryonic capacity for alpha function: for making meaning out of experience. This capacity enables the infant to make use of the mother and the mother's reverie.

When a life-threatening medical condition removes infants or young children from their mothers, there are a multitude of circumstances that impact the development of the contact barrier and create in the adult patient areas of psyche that are difficult to reach. Then adult traumas, most especially those found in everyday relationships, and certainly in the analytic relationship, provoke a return to infantile states of mind where, in extreme cases, the adult cannot be reached because he does not experience himself or the other. His contact barrier has been replaced by a wall of somatic perceptions, what Bion (1962) called a beta screen. The patient with a seemingly impenetrable beta screen loses his subjective sense of self. Instead there is a mental void (Lutenberg, 2007) or a black hole (Tustin, 1986; Grotstein, 1990). In those instances, the analyst must call forth the infant and receive the call to come forth herself.

This is true because the patient has retreated to a fused place of projecting out into the universe. This "place", which Teising (2005) calls the monadic and Ogden (1989a; 1989b) calls the autistic contiguous position, interferes with the patient's own subjectivity. Without a relationship to self, the patient loses contact with his or her own impulses and desires. Instead of love or hate as found in the Kleinian paranoid schizoid position, there is indifference. Indifference is difficult for any analyst. Indifference occurs when experience is flattened, so that everything carries the same weight, and is of equal importance—that is, unimportance. The resulting passivity makes relationships one-sided. It then appears that the only one in the relationship is the analyst and whatever is dealt with comes from her. The extreme passivity creates an impasse (Joseph, 1971; 1975). In some instances, the impasse comes with the first contact, whether by phone or in the office.

An example is a long-term patient, whom I will call Lazarus, with whom I worked first in psychotherapy and then in analysis for many years. He is a patient who taught me much and who had amazing courage to face the truths about himself. He also eventually became able to face truths about me. He taught me about myself as well, putting me up against my own horrors, terrors and retreats, up against my own limitations as well as my misunderstandings of theory.

Lazarus's trauma was two-fold. Reportedly, after three days of labor, the doctor came to his father and told him, "You have a monster baby. You will have to choose: Should I save the baby or the mother?" As the family myth goes, his father could not choose, and eventually the baby was born by caesarean. The mother and baby remained in hospital, separated from each other for several weeks. Both nearly died. Hence I say two traumas, one involving life and death issues physically, and the other involving life and death issues psychically.

My work with Lazarus also nearly died. Often, I felt we were getting nowhere. Just when something began to happen, he would interrupt his treatment. Even when he was present physically, I couldn't find him emotionally. Often I experienced myself as being "gone" to him, no matter that I was listening, responding and speaking. He seemed unaware that I was there. If I tried to speak to this, he retreated and was "gone" from me. I was left with myself and my observations and thinking. Since there were external changes in his life, I felt something important happened. We made contact with each other after he was able to connect with himself. That period of time was chaotic and painful for both of us. When his indifference began to break up, his idealization of me and denigration of himself made our work nearly impossible. When his idealization of me broke up, we began to be able to analyze his own grandiosity and infantile omnipotence. His alternate raging and suffering was awful for both of us. His grief seemed to go on and on. Still, during the last years of our work, he married; he gained professional success and recognition, which gave him financial stability. Better still, he left, grieving but happy, saying to me that he had found himself. He called me his Beatrice. I felt both of us had been through nine circles of hell and survived.

Tracing the differing kinds of silences in the years that Lazarus and I worked together demonstrates both a technique and a countertransference process of making contact with him in the hour and in the moment. Countertransference enables us to find our difficult to reach patients and to find ourselves. Some of this is noticing ourselves noticing them and noticing them noticing us. Noticing is important because, in order to mimic, noticing (Eekhoff, 2013) must take place. Noticing is not blankness. It is an impulse to connect. These patients get rid of that impulse too. One patient, who was better integrated, and therefore able to speak about it, called it "getting rid of the ridder". Lazarus often got rid of the ridder. In doing so, he appeared to be in limbo, and in fact it was this self-perception that ostensibly brought him to me.

Before focusing on silences, let me provide context. In the first session Lazarus told me he was desperate for a good therapy, but he had no money, earning only a subsistence living doing the odd consulting job. In what was then an uncharacteristic stance, I told him I was sorry he had no money but I could not treat him for free, or even for a reduced fee. He would have to find a way, and I would be happy to work with him. He said, "OK, I will come once a month." Again, I said, "No. I would only be taking your money and not helping you." He left, calling me several months later to come in, telling me he had found a job to pay for his therapy. I agreed to see him.

Initially he presented as a charming, handsome, intelligent man who was under-achieving. At 50, he had never been married, never held a job longer than a year in spite of a graduate degree. He told me he had a good year if he made $25,000. In spite of this, he moved in circles with the rich and famous and artistic. In our once a week session, which he paid for at the time and with cash, he told me story after story about his life. Although I found the stories interesting and somewhat entertaining, I was not moved by them, even as I had not been moved by his request for a low fee or a once a month treatment. I wondered about this, but in my inexperience felt it was something only about me. I did not then understand that his stories were walls of sound that kept us from making contact with each other. Rarely was there silence between us. Neither of us could tolerate it. His eye contact was good. His manner was polite and somewhat distant. His stories were articulate and at times amusing. His vocabulary was impressive. Still, I did not feel charmed or entertained. In truth, I did not feel much, something unusual for me. I carefully paid attention to my seeming indifference, analyzing myself to try to understand what was happening to me with my patient.

From the beginning, I could not find the meaning in his stories. Whenever I made an interpretation, he would politely listen, nod, agree and move on. I was left feeling how intelligent he was and how ignorant and uneducated I was. When the story returned again later, as it always did, it was obviously the same story I had heard before. Nothing had changed. He once said, "You must be getting tired of hearing the same thing over and over." The truth was that I was not, as I was so struck by his ability to tell the same story with the same words and inflections over and over again. Again, my feeling was that there must be some way he felt I did not hear him or did not understand. Perhaps my indifference to his stories bothered him. Yet my attempts to explore this were stopped, usually by being ignored. The exploration between us failed; however, I continued to explore inside myself, looking for the sources of my indifference. Also missing in these first months of our work together, as I said earlier, were silences.

I began to look for the slightest of changes in him or in me. When or if I noticed them I would say something about the change. Doing this had a surprising effect on him. He began to try to please me, elaborating his story, watching my face and proceeding or not, depending upon what he imagined he saw there. He seemed to be trying to find me now, as if I were not there. I began to feel useless and under scrutiny, but I had no sense that he felt anything. What I was feeling was about me, not yet about my patient, or so I thought. He did not complain about me. No matter how I interpreted the transference, he would politely deny any such thing. There were occasional silences. These had a quality I did not understand at the time. I thought he was using them to think. He was not. I thought he was waiting for me to say something else. Nor was he doing that. The silences appeared empty, which I had difficulty comprehending. The silences were dead. Later he said it was as if his mind stopped and was in suspension.

I came to realize, after more than a year of working with Lazarus, that I really did not exist as a person for him. When I told him this, he was surprised. He said, "I thought you knew that. Of course you are not here." I wondered aloud, as I had numerous times wondered silently, "You still keep coming for some unexplainable reason." He was silent. I too was silent. It seemed he was waiting for me to show up. He was looking at me looking at him looking at me, looking at ... Well, you get the picture. There really wasn't anything to say to that. Both of us seemed suspended in a hall of mirrors. We were two-dimensional reflections of each other, getting smaller and smaller into infinity.

The unconscious phantasies of both analyst and patient create an environment that may or may not result in both learning from experience (Bion, 1962; 1970). My horror at noticing myself absent to him soon became awareness that my patient also was gone. Both of us were suspended in limbo, awaiting a spontaneous gesture (Winnicott, 1971). In the waiting, I began to focus on my own or his impulse to speak. I noticed that the impulse to speak seemed to originate in the mind of one or both of us, not in any affective wish to communicate. In waiting, there could have been a silence that was productive and creative. Each of us might have been able to sense the other and receive projective identifications. Each one of us might have been able to stay present to ourselves and to each other. Then, when an impulse appeared, we might want to speak to the other, share our experience. In waiting, there were also many other possible kinds of silence. Some might have been hostile, some comfortable, some oppositional, some mixed. The silences between us, when we could tolerate them, were all of these plus another, more difficult silence.

The difficult silence was blank and empty. The blank silence seemed to have no impulses or thoughts in it. Since I believed this to be impossible, the blank silence horrified and terrified me. How could there be so little projection occurring in either direction? Since working with Lazarus, I have found this blank silence with other severely regressed patients and with schizoid patients. It occurs with psychotic or autistic patients. I since have found it exists with patients who might be called "as if" personalities (Deutsch, 1964). My patient did not appear to be any of these. He seemed to be primarily neurotic. Yet there was a mental void inside of him, a place where nothing seemed to be.

No wonder Lazarus and I both avoided silence. I believe now it was because of the horror we each experienced at recognizing the empty silence, of having no one and no thing present. Each of us had disappeared into infinity. The limbo was a frozen state where nothing could be learned and no one could be found. Instead of two people sitting across from each other, I became aware of sensations: sounds, images, smells and the minutest physical sensation. Initially, these somatic awarenesses seemed without meaning, merely defensive. It was as if I were suspended in time: quick-frozen. The action in the moment and in the session was of freezing sensate experience. Freezing meant that I became my environment. I became the background and blended with my patient. When I noticed this, it was possible to find words to describe something that was also true of him. When I spoke and became the foreground for Lazarus, I discovered ways in which he became like me, adopting my posture, my gestures, even my tone of voice if not my words. I noticed subtle mimicking. In accessing this awareness, I was able to think about it. There was an important relationship between us that I had previously been unable to detect.

The relationship was not about fight or flight, which involves an awareness of danger. It was not about survival. This relationship represented the infantile experience of relationship to the concrete sensations of the machines that kept him alive in the absence of his mother, before he had an awareness of danger. He related to me as an ever-present machine, or as a placenta, or as an absent mother. I believe such suspended limbo states occur naturally for all babies in utero, and even periodically for babies in the first three months of life. Infants separated at birth from their mothers have a frozen place that cannot be thought about or mediated where they are in limbo, waiting to be called into existence. When accessed in adulthood, this limbo state is the ultimate preverbal defense. It is an area of un-symbolized and unrepresented somatic experience.

Development continues when an infant's life is saved. Moms and babies reunite and babies develop physically and mentally. During an analytic process in search of the infantile transference, cognition continues. Emotion superficially develops. In the absence of drive and deep emotion, there is no impulse to act or to think. The psychic retreat that an analytic process uncovers is a time of clichéd speech or mimicry where emotional contact between two people is impossible. It is a time of stories, repeated word for word with the same inflection. These stories are hypnotic. This frozen in limbo state is more complicated than either imitation (Gadinni, 1969) or going through the motions because there is no awareness of it. Imitation comes later in development because in imitation there is a self who imitates and an "other" being imitated. In mimicry, it is as if the pause button has been pushed; yet in becoming the other, there is acknowledgement the other exists (Eekhoff, 2013; 2015).

Adult patients who have been separated from their mothers as infants seem to develop around a blank place where they do not psychically exist. In the silence of the couch, they at times do not find themselves. Without themselves, they experience the analyst as "not there". They feel nothing, so have no impulse to speak, no desire to do anything. These blank moments are extremely difficult for an analyst because it is tempting to attribute meaning that is not there, for example, resistance or aggression. Interpreting the aggressive or resistant level will only feed into a deep sense of shame for being somehow inadequate, without knowing why. The shame itself is diffuse, and cannot easily be attributed to either the patient or the therapist. Attributing meaning that is not there reinforces the defenses that have grown around the un-thought, but known, empty core. The blank place is not depression or resistance or even passivity, although it can look like all three. Nor is the blank place shameful. Shame is a later development. Analyzing the shame, while important, is a distraction from the blankness, the no place and the no person of the patient in the silence. Shame also may at least in part be the analyst's own narcissistic shame at not understanding or being confused.

I believe that this blank place interferes with many analyses because it is so pervasive. The blank place contributes to a feeling of having no floor for experience. If I do not realize that one or both of us has disappeared quietly from the room and into a black hole, I analyze what is developmentally at a higher level than the infantile transference of blankness. The analysis may become interesting and engaging, but it ultimately misses the underlying dynamic. Once this blank place has been accessed, the patient and the analyst must experience the horror of witnessing it, then the terror of embodying it and finally the rage over the loss. Only then can it be grieved. In grieving, symbolization can begin. All of this can only be accomplished in relationship. Because horror and terror and rage are unpleasant, one or both members of the treatment can flee. Sometimes it is obviously the patient who interrupts his treatment. In the hour, it is as often the analyst who cannot tolerate the intensity of nothingness and the horror and terror it evokes in her.

Back to Lazarus: Following his surprise that I had not known that I did not exist for him, I suggested working twice a week. He readily agreed. He was still sitting up. I began to look forward to seeing him, and decided this was evidence he was beginning to project, and to project positive feelings. When I interpreted this he denied it, apologetically. He told me it must be hard for me to work with him since he felt absolutely nothing for me. He found our sessions mildly interesting, he said, but they really did not change anything important about his character. His core was the same. He said he was the monster, unfeeling, uninterested and too much for this world. I became the one to care for him while he denied any feelings—either good or bad—about me. I was suffering and in labor. He was unable to be born. At the time, I did not know that. I only felt that I was failing.

I believe now that he was correct in that not much was changing at his core. Something was changing in the relationship, however. He had been seducing me and I was succumbing. Here was another impasse. I had become the needy baby and he the unavailable and unapproachable mother, who had everything. Of course, he matter-of-factly denied anything I said about him. He was mildly interested in knowing what I was experiencing. And, in a way, he seemed to be trying to take care of me. Silences were present as something almost titillating and mildly exciting, but mostly the silences yielded no insights and few interpretations. The transference had become perverse because the adult was hiding the baby who desperately needed a mommy analyst and was terrified. In the silences, I began to pay attention to his body and to mine, noticing and remarking on his breathing or his movement, attempting to mark and find meaning in his nonverbal presence.

About this time Lazarus began to talk about the women he was dating. Coincidentally I learned that he had had many therapies. Although he did not talk about his previous therapies, he did talk about what he called "my other women." There were always at least two, besides me. I learned about his history with women, of having sex with a fellow patient in a therapy group he was in, in spite of the rules of the group. They would have sex in the parking lot before and after therapy. He told me he did not initiate contact with women. They initiated contact with him and set the frame for the relationship. Sex was at their request. Since he was indifferent, not caring one way or another, he would have sex with them. He did not deceive them by making promises, or even by hiding his indifference or his other relationships. There was a feeling of perversion, of voyeurism I could not escape. What I might have called promiscuity was, to him, merely giving women what they wanted.

The promiscuity in the hour was found by the inability to attach to any thought or idea or emotion. One was as good as the next or the last. The silences implied that only my words were valuable. He was waiting for contact from me. He was indifferent to our attempts at understanding, but he seemed to cling to the sound of my voice and the rhythm of my speech. The perverse sexual excitement in the room was daunting. The silences became loaded with it. Yet it was difficult to speak to and get a response. I gradually sensed that I was in the room but he was not. I was an innocent watching a perverse pornographic film, where the sadist and the masochist changed roles continually. Again, I was horrified.

After some time, I came to realize that this was not an erotic transference in the classical sense. Instead, this was a transference of infantile polymorphous sexuality. Every interaction was exciting. It frightened me as I felt there was no escape from being myself in the room with him. He felt my interpretations as seductions. He felt my very presence as seduction, much as a plant is seduced by the light. My dread deepened. I could not find a way to speak to his infantile need that he could hear.

The next change in my countertransference happened so subtly; I still cannot say what it was. I only know that I began to dread seeing him. This was not just dread in the sessions, but dread of seeing him at all. For weeks, I would feel tense and withdrawn before our sessions. There was no longer any talk of other women, only talk now about his mother and how seductive she had been and how clinging and weak and demanding. He said his father was pretty much out of it, leaving him to care for her. I interpreted his feeling about my being seductive. "Who wouldn't like attention from a beautiful and wise woman?" was his reply.

When I interpreted the infantile transference in the here and now of the session, Lazarus would pause, cock his head and say, "Maybe." Usually he would say, "I do not have needs." Certainly, he did not seem to have needs. He reportedly lived in a small, barely furnished apartment. His needs seemed to be books and art. He was indifferent or passive about most things. The passivity I am talking about is having no desire at all. He seemingly felt no impulses of his own to do anything. Passivity without desire or impulse is also not about resistance or opposition. Resistance is something we analysts understand. This "no impulse" is more difficult to grasp. My experience of dread seemed to mark a break in his passivity and in the suspension of desire.

When I interpreted the dread he might feel about coming to see me, he would say, "It is so useless." My dread, I have since come to realize, covered over an intense horror. I was witnessing something I could barely hold in my mind, something so horrific as to be unbelievable. He was violently erasing himself over and over again, and somehow I was responsible because I allowed it or didn't get it or was indifferent to the violence he did to himself. It was not me who was absent in the room all these months, but him. Now that I knew it, I remained a helpless witness, almost as if he were a monk, burning himself alive in the midst of a crowd of "me's" who were helpless to stop him. Saying it aloud seemed to fan the flames.

When I suggested that he come three or four times a week and use the couch, he said, 'No." As much as I believed he needed analysis, I was pleased with his clear 'No". Maybe I was also relieved. I told him he had to find a way to find himself by opposing me. He told me he could not oppose someone who did not exist for him, who was a nothing inside of him. He thought I still did not get how unrelated he was to me or to anyone. I told him that I thought it was he who did not exist except as a mirror for me. He denied this also, but soon confirmed this by telling me I did not get how he annihilated himself over and over so that no experience could accumulate within him. He brought me a Winnicott article about this process the day that he told me he had accepted a job four hours away and would have to stop his therapy. I protested, told him we were just starting. He shrugged, said I was the one who told him to get a job, referring back to our very first session. I saw him two more times to say goodbye, and he was gone.

A year later, Lazarus telephoned and asked to come in. When I saw him he said nothing had changed, although he was making good money. He wondered if I would be willing to work with him again, after his precipitous leaving. He said he knew I had been right, that he shouldn't have left, and wondered aloud, "Don't analysts have ways of stopping people like me who do self-destructive things?" I interpreted his disappointment in our work and his anger at me for not being good enough for him. He said, "You still do not get that this has nothing to do with you. I am the monster." For over a year he commuted four hours twice a week to see me. His stories were more and more about his present life and relationships, or about what he was reading. He frequently quoted Shakespeare or talked about Dante's *Inferno*, quoting sections of it. He acknowledged his anger more often, although blamed himself for it. The silences were more frequent and we were able to speak about them, noticing their variety and differing meaning.

One day after being pleasant and chatty, he sat silent for several minutes. I too was silent. I was mostly waiting for him, looking out the window at the budding green trees, feeling relaxed and patient, occasionally looking at him. He too was mostly not looking at me, but seemed to be internal. Suddenly, I felt a very sharp pain in my chest. I very nearly gasped aloud with the pain. I couldn't breathe, so intense it was. I looked at him, fearing he had noticed. But he was looking out of the window, a serious expression on his face. The pain went away when I looked at him.

After a moment, he turned to me and told me he didn't know what his thoughts had to do with me or with our work together. He was silent again. Then he said he was remembering a *National Geographic* article about an Eskimo woman who had gone fishing with her infant and her two-year-old. The ice on which she was standing broke off and floated away from the mainland before she noticed. The three had lived for a while on raw fish and snow. No one found them. Slowly it occurred to her that they were going to die. Still she tried to live and keep her babies alive. She nursed her infant and her toddler, knowing she no longer had milk. She taught her toddler to chew leather. Then one day her baby bit her nipple. My patient's version said the baby bit the nipple off, something that hardly seems possible. Certainly in his phantasy it was true.

In my reception of Lazarus's unbearable fantasy, I felt the tearing of my own flesh, along with both horror and then fear. His story continued. The mother then strangled her baby and her toddler, throwing them into the sea. Her rescue from a patrolling coast guard boat came later, reportedly on the same day. My patient was silent, soundlessly weeping for the first time in our work together. I too was silent and wordless. No words came to me, only an unbearable physical pain in my body and then an overwhelming mix of indescribable emotions. Later, outside of the session, I felt fear and incredible grief. I sobbed after he left.

This event became the material for an exploration of our transference/countertransference relationship that moved between intellectual analysis of the back and forth of our process to emotional interactions with tears, anger and pounding the couch. Lazarus said he was afraid he was killing me. Then he feared that I would kill him. There simply could not be two of us alive at the same time. Often we would be silent for minutes at a time. I would attempt to process these silences, since no two of them felt the same. During one such silence, he told me he had been mostly blank but then an image of a chicken had popped into his mind. He said it was as if he were a chicken and I had a cleaver which I used to split apart his breast bone and rip out his heart. He tried again to leave his analysis, this time less successfully as he left for a month, using business travel as an excuse. When he returned, he was angry with me that I had not suggested that we talk on the phone while he was out of town.

Several months afterwards, he began to use the couch. Using the couch made a huge difference in our work together. Silence became a regular feature. I no longer felt so scrutinized or pinned down by his manners. I rarely felt the dread that had been pervasive for so long. Although he still maintained I was not there for him, he began to spontaneously free associate, something that had never happened before. He began to remember his dreams. Just as I was feeling our work was going well, in spite of my frequent confusion and doubt, he once again prepared to leave. This time he was thankful and grateful for our work, but said he thought it could go on forever. Some days as he prepared to leave he would tell me how disappointed he was in himself and in me that we could not go further. He said he knew it was not just his limitations but also mine. Still he was quite generous, saying he never thought we would get this far. He was no longer afraid of killing me, but he hoped not to take care of me in my old age as he had his mother. Now we had both reached our limitations. Again, after the session, I realized that we had reached the trauma of his birth and that he could not be born. One or both of us would die. He needed me to birth him and he was angry with me for failing.

Somewhere in this leaving came a remarkable session. The session before the remarkable one, Lazarus told me that I was just like his mother, weak and unable to take his intense emotion. He complained that if he did not have to take care of me, he would be able to get at his rage and murderous feelings. So, what good was it to stay with me anyway? I couldn't take it. I didn't know what to do, and he was just tormenting and punishing me session after session. He also accused me of clinging to him and making him feel guilty for wanting to leave. I remember attempting to interpret his fear that I would have to choose and would it be him, the monster, or me, the mother, who would die. When I said this, he was silent, seemed to be crying, and reached back with his hand to me. I momentarily took it.

In the session I am recalling, Lazarus came in and lay on the couch. He wiggled about a bit, shifting from side to side and then settled in, lying stiffly, as if in a coffin, on his back, arms crossed on his chest, legs stiff and straight. Then he did not move for 45 minutes. I watched him, silently. He did not speak. During this session, I felt every imaginable emotion. In spite of feeling unbelievingly cruel, I did not speak. I watched him, noticing the tension in his body, noticing how little his chest moved when he breathed. I felt that if I spoke, as my impulses told me to, I would be asking him to meet me, to take care of me, to follow my agenda. I do not know why he did not speak, but he did not. At the end of the hour when I told him "It is time," he rose, nodded without speaking and left.

Lazarus cancelled the next week's sessions. When he returned, he was furious with me. However, his anger and attack did not last long before he began to sob. He cried for a very long time, wordlessly, but this time with sounds. I nearly cried with him, so moved was I by his grief. Again, our silent session became the source of weeks of processing, of rages and recriminations, of tears and silences. I continued to interpret his need of me and his need of four times a week analysis. He admitted it was true, but could not imagine how it could happen. I asserted he needed to see me more often, not leave as he had been threatening for months. He said he knew that was true; it just seemed physically impossible. Perhaps he could call me. I agreed, so our compromise was that he would continue to come twice a week and on two other days call me.

The phone sessions were revelatory for me. The sensory deprivation, except for sound, enabled Lazarus to feel himself, much as a fetus in utero must be able to hear his mother's voice. He became able to express his disappointment in our work and in himself. Several times he was able to tell me he felt angry with me when we were not together. Finally it seemed that both he and I were present on the phone at the same time. It was harder to be in the room together at the same time. It seemed our physical presences were too much for him. The phone sessions seemed to enable a shift so both of us could tolerate the reality of the emotional and alive other. Still, more often than not, one or both of us would disappear.

Of course, on some level, the patient is always there and wants to be. He may work hard on these other levels, trying to reach something that has gone missing in him. When Lazarus told me I was not there, he was already changing. He could perceive something missing. Perhaps that something was the lost mother of infancy when hospitalization took the infant away from his mother. Perhaps too, I had surrendered to his internal fantasy world and become the lost mother of his infancy. I believe that whatever it was that changed in him was related to allowing myself to feel so lost and horrified by what I saw in the house of mirrors. My recognition of my own overwhelming awareness and non-existence enabled him to recognize his own absence. Later he would say to me, "There is no there, there," referring to himself. There were other comings and goings during the rest of his analysis. The ending phase was quite tumultuous. We revisited all of what I have described to you. When he left for good, both of us were sad and happy. In the years since, he has periodically contacted me, calling or sending a note to thank me and to tell me he is doing well. I am always glad to know.

Most of us have learned to continue to exist via the coming and going of our mothers' bodies and minds. Freud's (1920) imaginative understanding of his grandson's play with both a spool and thread, as well as playing peek-a-boo with himself in the mirror, gives us insight into the responses of certain patients who, like Freud's grandson, are able to "disappear themselves". However, some are not able to reappear themselves, and so for much of their lives remain hidden behind a sensory wall of experience that enables them to function via mimicry and to suffer minimally the "slings and arrows of outrageous fortune". By focusing on concrete sensory body experiences instead of emotional relationships with others, these patients have been absorbed by their own concrete sensations, their physical selves. They have also become absorbed by the workings of their own minds, having much intellectual understanding without finding emotional meaning. Lost inside their own mental activities, they do not experience themselves experiencing. They have lost an ability to see the emotional impact they have on themselves and others. In spite of this, they are able to describe and tell us about states they themselves do not understand. It is our task to remember them and make meaning of them.

Patients who are hard to reach due to early infantile or even conceivably prenatal trauma present some specific problems for therapists. Pathological mimicry (Eekhoff, 2016; 2019), the imitation of human speech (Paul, 1997) and passivity (Joseph, 1971) that alternates with reactivity are some of the silent manifestations of the difficulty. Reactivity can be particularly difficult because it is often silent and unspoken, especially in the initial stages of treatment, and results in prematurely leaving the analyst. These patients may be very concrete while brilliant in specialized areas. Patients who are hard to reach (Joseph, 1975) require a firm frame and clear expectations, as without them they become almost unbearably anxious and reactive. Their reactivity also changes the frame subtly, which frightens them even more. In spite of needing the firm frame, I find myself bending it sometimes, as I did when I agreed to phone sessions or holding my patient's hand (Ferenczi, 1928). The challenge for me is to hold the frame while keeping the patient.

Since these patients have difficulty with representation, they also have difficulty differentiating conscious processes from unconscious processing. They rarely reported dreams, as their imaging is inaccessible. After some years of analysis, they become aware of dreams that are sensory in nature. In their depths, and even in what seems like their everyday functioning, they are adept at being in the moment. However this being in the moment is different than what we typically think it to be. It is experience without a past or future. Time and space collapse. Without a sense of time or space, it is difficult for them to connect with their own desires, their own impulses, and hence their passivity.

Impulse comes from desire. Early trauma, which separates the infant from the mother at birth or within the first year or two of life, interferes with the meeting of impulse, desire and satisfaction. Instead of being met and contained, desire and impulse are frustrated. Instinctive need for maternal contact is frustrated. Frustration of the need for another promotes a shattering, which in turn interferes with an accumulated experience of learning and satisfaction (Bion, 1970). Impulses themselves become associated with trauma, which moves the external trauma of the lost mother to an internal trauma of the lost self. The intrapsychic structure becomes compromised. It is not only that the external is experienced as traumatic. Simultaneously, the impulses of the body and the desires of the mind implode, having nowhere to go, no one with whom to attach. The result is that the natural biological impulses for relationship, necessary for survival, themselves become threatening. There is a kindling effect where inside and outside are confused and both subject and object are temporarily lost.

Without a containing mother to help the infant identify himself, the subjective sense of self is frozen in time. The self becomes suspended (Meltzer, 1975; Eekhoff, 2017). Impulses and desires are lost, and the infant in the adult becomes passive and overly compliant, overly accepting, mimicking a relationship instead of having one. Mimicry is physical and somatic, and provides the infant and the infant in the adult proof of existence. This beginning of life makes analytic work with patients suffering from infantile trauma treatable.

Sometimes, mimicry is the most authentic response to others that these patients can master, in spite of the fact that it can contain mockery, hostility, contempt, rivalry and envy. Mimicry also is evidence of an inanimate mechanical defense. Since no two people are the same, the attempt at sameness evokes a mechanical non-human matching. It is this that produces the feeling of horror in the analyst who experiences being mimicked. The horror is being forced to witness and be used as an instrument of the patient's self-annihilation.

Mimicry can also contain admiration, curiosity, desire and agency. It is evidence of the earliest relationship and prenatal containment. When mimicry is observed, valued and interpreted, the analyst as other can occur. Mimicry is never perfect, and it is in the imperfections that the existence of the patient is discovered. The treatment becomes alive when the patient can tolerate more somatic experience and be found by the analyst. This over-adaptation includes identification with and becoming whoever one is with—whether or not the other person is aggressive. Perhaps identification with an aggressor (Ferenczi, 1933) includes identification with an absent mother, where absence was experienced as aggression.

The process of identification is extremely important here. It is not only that the absent mother is an aggressor; it is also that the instinctual aggression in the infant is not held or contained by the absent mother. In the subsequent shattering, unconscious phantasies are projected out into infinity and only partially contained by the environment. This projection is different from projective identification. It is not meant for communication; nor is it a by-product of splitting. To the analyst, it may appear that there is little or no projection or identification. The projection is so complete at this primitive level of the mind; there is only blankness and nothingness. The identification is with every living thing. The opposite is also true. The identification is with nothing living.

When projections go out into the world and the universe, instead of into a containing mother analyst, the patient becomes lost in space, projected into infinity. The patient becomes whoever she or he is with and whoever the other requires. The experience of a subjective self that remains constant across time and with differing others does not happen. Instead, the repeated emptying of self, occurring during massive projection into the universe, leaves the patient drained and lifeless. The person becomes a two-dimensional flat caricature, without a sense of interiority, or, as one patient defined herself, "a cartoon character." Later she described a friend as "not in her stories. She is outside of herself in the world. She is like a balloon with no air." After some moments of silence she said, "I am not even a flat balloon."

The simultaneous existence of multiple states of mind and being in both infant and mother can be severely impacted in the absence of the mother. The absence then impacts the infant by breaking down experience, not into related bits and pieces but into fractals that are seemingly unrelated. Life becomes a perpetually moving kaleidoscope, with the patient becoming shards of reflected light. Making deep emotional contact with such a patient is difficult. The other continuously becomes a different object; the self also is continuously a different subject. Relationship is lost, and with it the potential for symbolization destroyed. What remains is concrete, sensory and fixed. The infantile transference once discovered becomes Dante's Inferno.

What is lost is innocence as well as potential. Innocence allows for the spontaneous gesture of being. It is not just the reality that comes in too soon. It is also defenses that come in too soon, interfering with and inhibiting the impulse to learn, grow and develop. The self liquefies, evaporates without a container. Freezing appears as a defense against liquefying or evaporating. Freezing is a destruction of fluidity and a fear of the loss of cohesion. Tonic immobility is experienced as psychic immobility. Discrete particles exist outside of relationships. A person or object is experienced from moment to moment as a totally different one. It is not as if difference is erased, but that difference is so great as to be unrelated from one instance to the next. Subject and object are continually lost, not to be found or recognized again.

Space and time collapse, and what remains is blankness or absence or nothing. Tustin (1986) writes about this in her book about autistic defenses in neurotic patients. What is, is the lost mother of infancy as well as the lost infant of the adult patient in our office. The analytic task of interpreting the infantile transference, of speaking to unconscious processes and of interpreting the transference becomes difficult, as all three of these components are so lost to the patient. Relationship is a mental activity for them. It is not physical or emotional. The primary impulse that remains is the impulse to observe and mimic. Being a participant observer is lost to them. And yet, this is not all, for every infant was once contained; and when the infant and mother reconnect after hospitalization, every infant experiences some maternal containment that gets the alpha functioning again. The mother too experiences the infant calling her motherliness forth. It is this experience as well as the inborn life instinct that makes these patients treatable.

Lazarus struggled to comprehend this experience. He told me he was never the same person from day to day or moment to moment. Nor was I to him. He could trust no one, including himself. He feared that I would choose to believe only one part of him and never see the whole of him. He brought me out, engaged with me, entertained and provoked me. He forced me to keep looking for him, and to remember what I found and bring it back to him. When I despaired, he came out and got me. Together we found his lost infant and lost mother of infancy.

Our relationship changed both of us.

References

Bick, E. (1968). The experience of the skin in early object-relations. *International Journal of Psychoanalysis*, 49: 484–486.

Bion, W. (1962). *Learning from Experience*. Northvale, NJ: Jason Aronson, 1994.

Bion, W. (1970). *Attention and Interpretation*. Northvale, NJ: Jason Aronson, 1994.

Deutsch, H. (1964). Some clinical considerations of the ego ideal. *Journal of the American Psychoanalytic Association*, 12: 512–516.

Eekhoff, J.K. (2013). Infantile trauma, therapeutic impasses, and recovery, *American Journal of Psychoanalysis*, 73: 353–369.

Eekhoff, J.K. (2015). The silent transference: Clinical reflections on Ferenczi, Klein, and Bion, *Canadian Journal of Psychoanalysis*, 23: 57–73.

Eekhoff, J.K. (2016). Evocation: The analytic work of introjective identification. *American Journal of Psychoanalysis*, 76: 354–361.

Eekhoff, J.K. (2017). Finding a center of gravity via proximity with the analyst, *Engaging Primitive Anxieties of the Emerging Self: The Legacy of Frances Tustin*, H. Levine & D. Power (eds.). London: Karnac.

Eekhoff, J.K. (2019). *Trauma and Primitive Mental States: An Object Relations Perspective*. Abingdon: Routledge.

Ferenczi, S. (1928). The elasticity of psycho-analytical technique, *Final Contributions to the Problems and Methods of Psycho-Analysis*, M. Balint (ed.), trans. E. Mosbacher. London: Karnac, 1955.

Ferenczi, S. (1933), Confusion of tongues between adults and the child, *Final Contributions to the Problems and Methods of Psycho-Analysis*, M. Balint (ed.), trans. E. Mosbacher. London: Karnac, 1955, 156–167.

Freud, S. (1920). Beyond the pleasure principle. *Standard Edition 18*: 1–64.

Gadinni, E. (1969). On imitation. *International Journal of Psychoanalysis*, 50: 275–484.

Grotstein, J.S. (1990). The "black hole" as the basic psychotic experience: Some newer psychoanalytic and neuroscience perspectives on psychosis. *Journal of the American Academy of Psychoanalysis*, 18: 29–46.

Joseph, B. (1971). On passivity and aggression: Their interrelationship. *Psychic Equilibrium and Psychic Change: Selected Papers of Betty Joseph*, M. Feldman & E.B. Spillius (eds.). London & New York: Tavistock/Routledge, 1989.

Joseph, B. (1975). The patient who is difficult to reach. *Psychic Equilibrium and Psychic Change: Selected Papers of Betty Joseph*, M. Feldman & E.B. Spillius (eds.). London & New York: Tavistock/Routledge, 1989.

Lutenberg, J.M. (2007). Mental void and the borderline patient. *Resonance of Suffering: Countertransference in Non-Neurotic Structures*, A. Green (ed.). London: Karnac.

Meltzer, D. (1975). *Explorations in Autism: A Psychoanalytic Study*. New York: Karnac.

Ogden, T.H. (1989a). *The Primitive Edge of Experience.* Northvale, NJ: Jason Aronson.

Ogden, T.H. (1989b). On the concept of an autistic-contiguous position. *International Journal of Psychoanalysis,* 70: 127–140.

Paul, M. (1997). *Before We Were Young: An Exploration of Primordial States of Mind.* Binghampton, NY: ESF Publishers.

Tustin, F. (1986). *Autistic Barriers in Neurotic Patients.* New Haven, CT: Yale University Press.

Teising, M. (2005). Permeability and demarcation in the psychoanalytic process: Functions of the contact-barrier. *International Journal of Psychoanalysis,* 86: 1627–1644.

Winnicott, D.W. (1971). *Playing and Reality.* London: Tavistock.

Part II

Embodied assaults

Chapter 5

When life intrudes

Experience of trauma in the body

Maureen Murphy

Introduction

Some years ago at an American Psychological Association (APA) meeting, I went to listen to a Division 39-sponsored panel entitled "Use of the Psychoanalytic Space". One speaker told the following story. He said:

> About 18 months into the analysis of a 37-year-old man, the patient was diagnosed as having testicular cancer. Between the time of the biopsy and the surgery, which took about a month, the patient was totally preoccupied with this issue. He was completely absorbed with concerns about whether he would live or die, his two young sons, and enumerable medical details. The patient was either disinterested in, or incapable of, examining fantasies and responded blankly to transference interpretations. The analyst felt it would be sadistic, even if accurate, to confront the patient's avoidance of these topics, and felt at a loss about what to do. Since no real analysis was possible during this period, he wondered if he should carry on with supportive psychotherapy or perhaps suggest that they interrupt treatment until the surgery was over and, hopefully, recovery was underway.

Having become engrossed in the story, I was totally unprepared for the analyst's comment about the impossibility of analysis at this point, and horrified at even the consideration that treatment would be suspended. After the remaining speakers finished, an impassioned audience discussion ensued, entirely focused on this vignette crystallizing the question: Does psychoanalysis have anything to offer during an actual trauma? The discussion took the turn you might imagine—that our theoretical understanding of what constitutes analysis would ultimately inform our intervention. I left comforted by the thought of other, though unspecified, technical options.

I came to psychology with my professional experience as an intensive care nurse dealing with children undergoing open-heart surgery. My work mainly involved preparing my young patients and their parents for this experience.

There was a simulated room with all of the accoutrements of the actual ICU in which the children could play and rehearse the events of the days to come. The idea was that some passing familiarity would diminish their terror on waking from anesthesia and hasten, or at least not impede, their recovery. Similarly, by orienting parents beforehand, it was hoped that they would be more available to the child postoperatively. While all of this helped, it soon became clear, especially for the parents, that talking about how they felt was the most effective way of keeping them available to their children. So, when I entered graduate school it was with the expectation that I would integrate psychology with my continuing work in health care. Instead, as I became engrossed in psychoanalysis and the demands of clinical training and practice, my original plans receded.

Given this path to psychology, it has always been surprising to me to hear that psychoanalysis has little to offer people during an illness, or indeed during any actual trauma. After a latency of nearly 30 years, a parallel set of experiences required me to grapple, once again, with the question that first brought me here. In my professional life I was confronted with two sets of patients being diagnosed with cancer which coincided with my husband's life-threatening cardiac illness. Both personally and professionally, I was plunged back into the gray zone where mind and body intersect palpably, where the boundaries between being a therapist and a witness blur, and where words are hardly above a whisper.

In this chapter I attempt to delineate what contribution psychoanalysis can make to a situation in which actual events fundamentally disrupt lives. In the first part I describe the subjective experience of trauma drawn from my therapeutic relationships as well as personal anecdotes. Second, I propose a theoretical understanding of those experiences; and, finally, I conclude with some implications for practice in dealing with these patients and their families.

The subjective experience of trauma

In his work with holocaust survivors and their families, Krystal (1985) identifies three hallmarks of development most assaulted by trauma: differentiation, verbalization and de-somatization.

Differentiation refers to the development and maintenance of those boundaries which separate self from non-self. In the earliest days of development, the mother serves as an environmental barrier to insulate the infant from everyday, yet overwhelming, stimuli. She is assisted in this task by the somatic integrity of the infant, notably the skin, and by numerous soothing ministrations that protect the baby from premature collision with distress. When these internal functions are adequate, the subjective experience of the baby is one of safety and cohesion. Where differentiation has been successful, the individual has been able to transform global anxiety into manageable pieces, or nameless dread into defensive strategies.

In trauma, this cohesion stands in contrast to feelings of falling, shattering and fragmenting. Experiences are split into sensations—impressions—rather than being integrated into perceptions. Perception encompasses our usual mode of everyday life: logical thought, secondary process, temporal-spatial dimensionality. When there is an atomizing of sensation and perception in the direction of sensation, all of the structures that support a sense of me-not-me are compromised.

What defies time and space defies logical and symbolic thinking threatening the usual landscape of psychoanalysis.

Perhaps the main vehicle of differentiation is verbalization. From the initial murmurings and mutual cooing to specific naming, a nearly unbroken sound tapestry binds caretakers and children. Paired with physical contact, language sorts out stimuli with increasing specificity. Gaddini (1987) calls the acquisition of language "consolers"—consolation for the loss of the original mother–infant dyad. The mouth now trades sucking for word-making. The acquisition of language underwrites the capacity to symbolize, and draws the person into an increasingly causal, less random, safer world. Verbalization acts to sustain differentiation, foster autonomy, and facilitate individuation.

Along with differentiation and verbalization comes a gradual emergence from life in and as a body. Language permits de-somatization by providing another means of attaining satisfaction. Physical development paradoxically serves de-somatization as the body progressively becomes the servant rather than the master. Cognitive development likewise weakens bodily dominance in favor of interpersonal negotiation.

When trauma occurs, this triad is disrupted and replaced by modes of functioning so unfamiliar that a new language must be constructed in order to preserve relatedness. How are these bastions of development destabilized?

Let me first introduce my patients. Already I have begun the process of dedifferentiation: "My patients". This is so commonplace as to be invisible and, in fact, is meant to convey an intimate connection between us. Yet these vestiges of de-differentiation are at once as essential to intimacy as to its corruption.

Mr. R, 55, was diagnosed with a rare breast cancer five years ago. At that time our treatment was of many years duration, two to three times a week. A radical mastectomy was performed, and his recovery proceeded uneventfully, as might be expected of an otherwise healthy person. About 18 months later, bilateral lung nodes appeared. Rather than attempt a biopsy, his doctor prescribed the drug Tamoxifen, an estrogen modulator used to treat breast cancer in men and women. This began an agonizing period of wait and see. Like prisoners of war and others in situations where their lives could be ended in a moment, patients with protracted illnesses personify time. A phenomenon that was full of potential and metaphor takes on causal significance encroaching on differentiation—what the poet Donald Hall (1996) calls time without punctuation. The Tamoxifen shrank the nodules, and last summer an elated Mr. R went off on a fitness retreat for two weeks of strenuous hiking. Shortly after his return, he fell bending down and was unable to get up. The metastasis had invaded his bones. Since then he has endured excruciating pain, chemotherapy and radiation. He has lost his hair; he can't drive or travel; his appetite has gone, along with his ability to savor his large wine collection. Nevertheless, he is militant about continuing his treatment, insisting on keeping our arrangements the same as much as possible.

When Ms. S was diagnosed with breast cancer, she underwent bilateral mastectomies (both breasts were malignant). The loss of her breasts was especially traumatic as she had been born without a uterus, something that had occupied us during her previous four years of treatment. The loss of her breasts robbed Ms. S of her one remaining confirmation of femininity. Post-operatively, Ms. S was treated with chemo and Tamoxifen, which in women precipitates immediate menopause. Her recovery has so far been excellent; yet, at the year anniversary of completing chemo, she began smoking.

From the personal perspective, my husband, Terry, suddenly underwent unsuccessful bypass surgery, which led to a heart transplant. While all life-threatening illness poses a threat to the self-fabric of any individual, the response elicited by a transplant goes beyond that of conventional medical procedures. The heart, romanticized as the home of the soul and wellspring of human relationship, takes on mythic proportions not found with other transplanted organs. Receiving the heart of another evokes a range of fantasies, from being a murderer to having a secret other—a Secret Sharer that even Joseph Conrad could barely have imagined. Here I was not the therapist; but I was also not *not* the therapist. I was always the witness, and, like all witnesses, the voice of what was or had happened. As one patient described this, "You have to be the memory machine." I found myself acting like a nurse, remembering obscure blood levels I hadn't considered for years. The staff readily treated me like a fellow professional, a refuge I gratefully accepted. It was a known reality to be a nurse—there is a language to speak, there is something quantifiable to do, all preferable to rampant anxiety, intrusion, numbness.

Now to the experiences. The erosion of differentiation and verbalization leading to resomatization during hospitalization has been amply documented. There are the well-known caricatures of "It's time to take our pills now, Mr. Jones." The crux of the matter is this: In the course of a protracted illness, an individual becomes involved in close, life-sustaining relationships with virtual strangers who relate through and about the body (as if it were the person), speaking in mechanical (non-symbolic) language about the unspeakable. This sense of our material body as a unit differentiating us from others is so established in adults as to be imperceptible. We rarely think about it or notice it except for being jostled in line or packed in an elevator. Nonetheless, our reliance on body-boundedness is profound. During various forms of physical trauma, the body is handled, pierced, in fact surrendered or expropriated in ways that compromise the most essential boundary.

Other important boundaries are similarly affected. Sitting in the waiting room of the chemotherapy department, your profession, whether you are a parent or not, that you have been a committed social activist, or the many other individual ways that we have constructed to give meaning to our lives are irrelevant. You become a cancer patient, or a transplant patient, or are here for a biopsy. These groups offer a peculiar boundedness that is at once embracing yet faceless. Such groups are often differentiated only by unique somatic circumstances. In this sense, to be included perpetuates de-differentiation and resomatization.

As boundaries are compromised, other structures assume critical importance. These are structures that we think of as the small weave, repetitive patterns that are often taken for granted. For example, when Mr. R first experienced bone metastasis, he was in considerable pain and had great difficulty walking. To get to my office requires climbing a steep set of stairs. He called to tell me that he would be unable to come to our sessions for a week, saying: "I feel panicked that I can't keep our appointment—I need to come in more than ever." Knowing that it could be more than a week before he would be able to navigate the stairs, I suggested that in the meantime we could speak on the phone. He said: "No, I want to see you." I offered to see him at his home if he wished. He said there wouldn't be enough privacy. When he was able to come into the office (in fact it was a week later) he said: "I really appreciate your offer to talk on the phone or come to the house, but I have to be here—I have to sit in this chair, then I can feel safe." Some months later when his hearing was temporarily impaired by radiation to his head, he said: "You'll have to come closer so I can hear you." I started to move a light desk chair towards him, but he protested that our usual upholstered chair should be moved. It was imperative that this aspect of the form be reliably preserved. With the loss of other external features, familiar shapes and forms take their place.

The destruction of language in trauma is the result of a reciprocal between the unthinkable and the unsayable. As an example, prior to my husband's transplant, I was asked the following question by loving, well-intended friends, many of whom have some connection to health care. They asked: "Where do the hearts come from?" The form of the question, and often the tone of voice, had the ring of the childhood query: "Where do babies come from?" Surely, they knew where the hearts came from. The question reflected the near impossibility of genuine thought about the meaning of transplantation and the concomitant difficulty speaking of it.

Especially to people who have been verbal in their pre-traumatic life, the compromise of language is particularly terrifying. At the same time, to speak of the reality of their circumstances is even more overwhelming. When my husband had the bypass surgery that presaged the transplant, everyone expected that it would go smoothly since bypass is now such a common procedure. This didn't happen. During the three weeks that Terry was in the ICU, I was in the hospital for 18–24 hours a day. After four or five days, my descriptions to friends and family began to sound hollow. I would hear myself saying: "This is a nightmare," yet feel like the language didn't touch my experience. Still reasonably calm, I decided to keep a daily journal where I could at least write what I actually felt. This was even less effective. The words evaporated as they took shape. I could see the words on paper, but they were written in an affectively invisible ink. I became increasingly panicked at the prospect of being cut off from language as a vehicle of connection. As a last resort, I began walking in the park across the street for long periods of time. After a few minutes of uninterrupted stride, I felt calmer, more optimistic. The sensation of sun or the fragrance of flowers was reassuring at a visceral level. No distress could be tolerated. If it was a windy day, I had to find a protected interior route; if it was too warm, I instinctively headed for shade. External impingements that interfered with a steady, predictable cadence were avoided at all costs. After these periods of respite, I could return to the details of the moment.

My patients and my husband were not so able to move between states of demand and withdrawal. They described a profound loneliness that is the result of a failure to symbolize and represent internal objects. The breakdown in connectedness to internal objects leaves the person excruciatingly lonely. The loneliness was characterized by the progressive loss of versions of creativity; interest in external events waned and the capacity to read was particularly terrifying. One patient, who belonged to a semi-professional chorus for 20 years before his transplant said: "I'll know I have survived when I can sing from my heart again—well, from somebody's heart." While in this state the patients would ask: "What has become of me?" and "Will I ever get my life back?" They were able to recognize their disconnection, yet unable to act on their own behalf to re-establish connection. Terry's journal chronicled this:

> I fight each day to stay emotionally even. There are so many "used to be's" in my life—so many that I am very worried that after the operation, the real person who has gone away, someone I truly liked on most occasions … will not return. One of my greatest fears is that I will grow so far away from who I was that it will be impossible to grow back.

Two particular features of verbalization illustrate the effects of trauma on language. First, Krystal (1985) and Laub & Auerhahn (1993) have described a tendency among Holocaust survivors to adopt condensed, somewhat childlike phrases to describe their experiences. In response to questions about the Holocaust, they might say repetitively: "They were all wiped out" or "The whole family is gone." Clearly such responses are intended to make the experience manageable in concept and in words at however elemental a level. Similarly, patients with physical trauma fix on a phrase to convey the totality of their experiences. Often it took the form: "I wouldn't be alive if it weren't for Sally." Sally (or whoever) is the person they have designated as the keeper of their aliveness. Usually, everyone familiar with the patient agrees that Sally does serve this function; yet it is remarkably devoid of the inter-subjective component we have come to expect in relatedness. I believe this is a clear example in adult life of Winnicott's (1969) concept of object use, as well as Ogden's (1991a) notion of the autistic-contiguous position.

The other feature of verbalization is the repetition of key phrases. Continuing with the previous example, Mr. R might say "I wouldn't be alive if it weren't for Sally" to me several times in a given session. I think of this behavior like the closing scene of Ray Bradbury's *Fahrenheit 451*, where the characters endlessly repeat verbatim the text of their favorite books after the fire as a way of preserving them. The repetition is self-soothing and safety-generating. There is another who is my mind now, relieving me of both thought and speech. The following clinical example illustrates this dynamic.

After her surgery, Ms. S received a year of monthly chemotherapy treatments. At their conclusion, Ms. S began to smoke—something she had never done before. I learned about it obliquely, when she was speaking about being forgetful as a side-effect of her medication.

She commented: "And I even left my wallet at the gas station where I stopped for cigarettes. "Cigarettes!" I blurted out. She looked at me blankly as if to say, "Surely you already knew this," and finally she told me she only buys them after leaving our sessions, smokes three or four and then throws them away. I felt such a jumble of affects that I couldn't formulate a sentence. Realizing this, I said: "Perhaps there is some outrage you want me to say on your behalf."

Ms. S: I am very worried about what will happen to me now that the chemo is over.

MM: It feels like the chemo has kept you alive and now that it's finished, how will you stay alive?

Ms. S: If I could have done it on my own, maybe I wouldn't have gotten cancer in the first place. I had a dream that I was dying. I was in bed and people gathered around. You sat close to me and held my hand, I thought, "If I am dying, Maureen will hold on to me."

MM: Now that you are not in danger of dying anymore, I might leave you to your own devices.

Ms. S: I know I have to start believing that I can take care of myself, keep myself alive, but I am not sure that I can do it yet. Buying cigarettes when I leave your office is like saying, "I can still die if you don't take care of me." Is this really me speaking?

This sequence illustrates two frequently occurring clinical issues. First, Ms. S is surprised that I didn't know about her smoking, since I had temporarily become her mind. Then she alludes to the unthinkable idea that no matter what she does, she could have a recurrence of her cancer. Her only hope of staying alive is to have me look out for her, providing the safety she can't provide for herself.

The subjective experience of actual trauma involves a breakdown of differentiation in terms of body boundaries, life in the external world, perception of time and the capacity for mutuality. The enormity of the insult robs the person of their capacity to think and the words to find their way out. The body once again becomes the main vehicle for relatedness; however this time, unlike the progression of the infant, the body becomes a prisoner delegating an external other to keep them alive until their sentence is served.

Theoretical considerations

A review of the trauma literature yields consensus that the main dynamic features could be summed up as: "A time lived through but not experienced as part of the self" (Cohen, 1985, p. 178). Each person has a personal narrative that is part of a reciprocal process of making meaning out of experience, an evolution of our earliest experiences of going on being. When confronted with experiences so overwhelming—devastating, shattering—that the mediating function of the ego is disabled, experiences cannot be cohesively inscribed in memory and are registered, instead, as massive arousal without the capacity for discharge. The individual is confronted with a situation in which he or she is "resourcelessly dependent" (Khan, 1972).

Because trauma interrupts the sense of going on being, it is experienced as the psychic equivalent of maternal abandonment—the rending of a dependable matrix. This matrix is known by various names: potential space, stimulus barrier—all holding environments enabling the progressive emergence out of a somatic cocoon. When there is an assault to this holding environment, the personal narrative by which we recognize ourselves—the continuing representation of a good object—is jeopardized. Kirshner proposes that it is the concept of the loss of the function of the good object that underwrites the common ground for psychoanalytic understanding of trauma. As Kirshner so felicitously puts it: "the good object is the premise and promise of the symbolic order" (1994, p. 239)—the order that is so profoundly disrupted in trauma.

Violation of the stimulus barrier results in an incapacity to organize memory in the service of forming internal representations. This failure eliminates the use of signal anxiety leading to the establishment of primitive, self-protective mechanisms aimed at minimizing or controlling the stimuli that evoked the trauma in the first place. Cohen and Kinston's work on primal repression (1985, 1986) and Ogden's concept of personal isolation (1991b), an elaboration of the autistic-contiguous position, are useful in charting this landscape. Their work attempts to account for those periods throughout life when individuals retreat from genuine relatedness in the face of unbearable experience. These states, essential to survival, alternate with more organized modes of existence usually characteristic of adult functioning.

As a way of grappling with clinical phenomenon reflecting failure to symbolize as opposed to repressed material, Kinston and Cohen posit the idea of primal repression. Repression, the cornerstone of classical psychoanalysis, does not usefully explain states in which there is an absence of representation. They describe primal repression as follows: "[P]rimal repression refers to an absence of psychic structure, that is to say of emotional understanding, where such structure could and should be" (1986, p. 338). The absence or loss of structure was brought about by traumatic events which left instead some form of permanent impression on the mind which is not usable or useful. Because the impression is not a representation (in the usual sense of that term), it does not require specific mental activity to keep it from consciousness. However its presence manifests powerfully in a person's relationships and leads to reproduction of the trauma or aspects of it throughout his life. Cohen (1985) conceptualizes primal repression as a stage of development prior to repression proper, but which can be re-evoked at any developmental point in the presence of significant trauma, physical or psychological. Clinically such states, which they call "holes", are "conveyed by pre-representational, experiential elements including sensory impressions, stereotyped actions, physiological reactions and isolated images or affects" (pp. 180–181). Cohen proposes that primal repression characterizes all psychopathology. In severe psychopathology, as in actual trauma, this is the predominant mode of existence. In this connection these authors make what I believe to be a central contribution when they point out that in such severely compromised states the individual protects himself by primitive mechanisms, not ego defenses. The compromise formations accompanying defenses are absent. Instead these mechanisms protect by producing the opposite effect, namely that "symbolization and internalization are unreliable, relationships can't be deeply satisfying, and creativity is impoverished" (Cohen, 1985, p. 183). So in this sense these mechanisms eliminate pathways that would make possible thinking and saying except "through interactions with need-mediating objects" (p. 180).

Ogden's theory of the autistic-contiguous position extended the original Kleinian formulation to include this pre-symbolic level of experience. The autistic-contiguous position is associated with a mode of generating experience that is of a sensation-dominated sort and is characterized by protosymbolic impressions of sensory experiences that help to constitute an experience of bounded surface. Rhythmicity and experiences of sensory contiguity (especially of the skin surface) contribute to an elemental sense of continuity overtime (1991a, p. 595). The examples with Mr. R's insistence on being in the same room and chair illustrate adult versions of this position.

Elaboration of the autistic-contiguous position gives definition to Cohen's notion of holes in the personality. Holes in this sense are islands of experience embroidered with impressions of hardness or softness covered with relatedness, yet not accessible to structural knowing. In severe psychopathology they cripple the personality. During periods of trauma they can riddle a previously intact psyche temporarily or more ominously, depending on the degree of the assault.

Ogden has also used the concept of "personal isolation" to describe a phenomenon incorporating the autistic mode of generating experience. He describes personal isolation as a refuge "against the continuous strain that is an inescapable part of living in the unpredictable matrix of human object relations" (1991b, p. 385). The subtitle of Ogden's article, "A Breakdown of Subjectivity and Intersubjectivity," implies the consequence of a retreat so pervasive that it forecloses intra-personal as well as interpersonal connectedness. In a world of personal isolation the individual lives by autistic shapes and forms. Shapes convey sensations and forms convey boundedness. Both vectors have an orienting function that preserves relatedness, albeit at a primitive level. In such a mode the burden of relationship falls heavily on the other. As Cohen says of analytic experiences in this mode: "These often hang loosely together and do not usually lead to a well-formed understanding in the analyst's mind that can be usefully feedback as an interpretation" (1985, p. 178). Ogden likens the experience of the analyst with such a patient to the mother who must allow her infant his own periodic sanctuary and tolerate her own temporary nonexistence. In order for the relationship to survive, however, the mother/analyst must be able to successfully "compete" and retrieve the infant/patient.

Shortly after my husband's transplant surgery, he was still hovering between consciousness and unconsciousness. For the first 24 hours his physicians thought he was best left undisturbed. On the second day when his physician arrived for rounds he was distressed to learn that Terry would respond to requests to do this or that, but would not initiate contact. He approached Terry and said: "Terry, it's Ernie. I know you're in there. Come on out, I miss talking to you." Terry became alert and smiled, looking like somebody thoroughly rested. He even reached out offering to shake hands. The nurse was amazed and began to try to talk with him, but as soon as Ernie left, he again withdrew. Ernie's familiar voice and insistence on re-establishing their previous connection was compelling to Terry in a way that even the most benign pressure for a response to a caring, though unfamiliar, person could not be reciprocated. This vignette illustrates Ogden's view on the functions of personal isolation: "That uncertainty and unpredictability are suspended, and survival protected, by a shift in the balance of co-existing forms of being" (1991b, p. 385).

During periods of catastrophic trauma, times that are unthinkable and unspeakable, symbolic representations are forfeited and replaced either by withdrawal or reliance on the familiar at the level of sensation, not perception. The transference and countertransference elicited at these points in treatment require a stamina not usually asked of us. If, as was the case with my patients, we have a relationship of long standing, we must bear the temporary loss of that familiar interaction, while providing the patient almost unwavering steadiness.

The experience of treatment

Trauma is not a monolithic structure. How the effects are manifested by each person varies according to the nature and severity of the assault, as well as the duration. Returning to my patients, although Ms. S's illness involved mutilation and a potentially fatal outcome, her recovery has been smooth. Now, at just past two years, she remains free of metastasis. Mr. R, however, has been in this struggle for nearly five years, having most recently experienced brain metastasis. The depth and frequency of his withdrawal are more pronounced. These variations have a profound effect on both the treatment and the subjective experience of the analyst.

In this section, I describe the therapist's subjective experience of treatment, specifically feelings of loss by actual death, loss of the rich symbolic collaboration and, most confusingly, of getting lost in an explosion of projections.

In an article entitled "Personality Death, Object Loss, and the Uncanny" Feigelson movingly describes the experience of family members dealing with sudden brain damage to their spouses and parents. She characterizes the alive but damaged person as bearing an uncanny resemblance to their former self—familiar and unfamiliar at the same time. The family, whom she calls witnesses, bears the burden of relating to this alter-ego while coping with the living loss of their beloved. Feigelson describes three aspects of this strenuous task:

> First, the bifurcated object acts on the observer in a real sense. Second, the damaged person attracts (elicits in the witness) projected elements of early representations. Third, this alter-ego at the same time invites the projected, unwanted self-representations of the witness. (1993, p. 342)

While existence in a state of personal isolation that I have been describing is not synonymous with personality death, I believe the effect on the therapist is similar. When, as in the cases I have cited, the therapist has had a lengthy, intense relationship with a patient, the literal loss of their life is jangling to the therapist. All therapeutic work is an investment in the future, which is now clouded. For the therapist the death of the patient is also unthinkable.

When Mr. R first experienced bone metastasis, as I mentioned earlier, he fell and could not get up. He assumed this was an orthopedic injury due to over-exercising on his fitness vacation. He called to ask if we could reschedule, telling me the story and his presumed diagnoses. As he spoke, I felt nauseated and dizzy. In spite of the somatic alarm, I didn't register what I knew to be the more likely explanation. The night before I was next to see Mr. R, I dreamt that I had breast cancer. I awoke feeling anxious, still not making the connection. As Mr. R limped down the hall to my office, I suddenly recalled my dream. He sat down and gave a thumbs down signal and said: "You knew, didn't you?" I answered him honestly that I had been holding out for his version as much as he had.

In addition to the potential death of a patient, there is the loss of the usual mode of relating. Verbal symbolic interpretations have little currency with a patient operating at an autosensuous level. The therapist "competes" for the patient just as the environmental mother competes for her infant, relying on tone of voice, gestures and recollections of shared experiences. Yet there is the constant background nagging: "Is this therapy? Or am I really doing case management?" In Winnicottian terms, the environmental mother ideally remains unnoticed to both mother and baby, but here that role feels all too noticeable.

The autistic-related balance is a precarious one. When Ms. S underwent exploratory surgery which would terminate in mastectomy if malignant cells were found, I had to be out of town. We had agreed that I would call her at the hospital. When she returned to therapy she said that she had felt upset that I had called. This puzzled her, since she had longed for contact with me outside of treatment, a subject that we had explored many times. I felt initially stunned by her response, and also puzzled. We examined this topic a number of times with little success. When she approached her two-year anniversary, which included a full-body CAT scan, she experienced many of the same anxieties that she had during the initial diagnostic period. After receiving a clean bill of health, she left me a message with the good news. At our next session she told me:

> I wanted to call you right away. At the same time I had this feeling of dread. I hoped you wouldn't call me. I know we have talked about this a dozen times. Usually I spend all my energy just trying to find ways to run into you on the street. It finally occurred to me that when I was diagnosed I needed absolutely nothing to change; that included your staying on some unreachable pedestal. If you were human too, I was sunk.

Dealing with a sense of loss to the relationship as it had existed in the patient/therapist dyad serves as a model for the therapeutic task of helping the isolated patient remain connected to his or her family. In the cases I have described, as well as others I have treated, this parameter of involvement with other people in the patient's life regularly occurs. In situations in which there was no ongoing relationship, contact with the family regarding the previous level of functioning provides the necessary background material with which to construct meaning. I see this as an unusual, yet essential, function for the therapist in providing a footbridge between the patient and his or her increasingly dismayed family. Speaking for a patient who cannot speak for him or herself protects the connection between the patient and his or her object world. When Mr. R asked me if his fiancée could call me, I asked what he would like me to do. He replied: "Just say whatever will help her not be so scared." After we had spoken a few times, Mr. R said: "It is a relief to have you speak to Sally. I can see her pain, but I can't find any words. I just feel blank."

As Feigelson suggests, mutual projections characterize the relationship with traumatized individuals. The therapist's own primitive fears are re-ignited with the potential of being projected onto the patient. A patient who had been a victim of a horrible crime was referred to a therapist immediately following the attack. As she told her story, the therapist fell asleep. I believe that listening to the violent details of this patient's assault was unbearable—the therapist escaped into sleep. The patient came away believing literally that nobody wanted to hear about her experience and that to speak of it would certainly drive people away. On the other hand, awareness of these projections is the most useful (often the only) way to remain in contact with the patient. One day when a technician came to draw yet another blood sample from my husband, I strangled the urge to scream "Don't touch him!" After the technician left I commented to Terry that he tolerated all of these tests amazingly well. He replied: "It might look like that, but I really felt like, 'Don't touch me, you bastard.'" In an article by Elizabeth Lloyd Mayer (1994) about an analysis she conducted with a dying patient, Mayer says that in this analysis she allowed herself to be "ruthless and inspirational." These are words found little enough in psychoanalytic case presentations, especially when used to describe technique. Nonetheless, I thought of them as quite accurate, but from a different vantage point. With traumatized patients the analyst experiences the ruthlessness of these primitive states of isolation with all of the valence of Winnicott's meaning. In turn, the analyst "competes" for the patient with various gestures that inspire, or at least preserve, relatedness. The analyst finds the lost words, returns them to the patient in a way that promotes cohesion out of chaos, like all witnesses, the voice of what was or had happened.

Let's return to the question of whether psychoanalysis has anything to offer in periods of acute trauma. Regardless of internal theoretical disputes, psychoanalysis is essentially a theory of development in the context of meaning. The major contribution of contemporary theorists has been an awareness of the endurance of the primitive edge of experience throughout life in all types of personalities. During periods of trauma we see this edge more clearly and pervasively than usual. We hold out to patients the possibility of a nuanced understanding of the fabric of their lives as it is dialectically constructed by material and immaterial experience. In this sense collaborating with a person objectively in acute trauma and subjectively on the threshold between meaning and oblivion is the bargain we made in the first place.

We can also ask the question of whether the psychoanalyst has anything to offer in periods of acute trauma—particularly when operating somewhat beyond the rigor of theory and typical psychoanalytic practice. For the therapist, primitive images of body parts, feeling lost, falling, not being able to get up, torn skin, no hair provoke anxiety and the impulse to turn away. These unwanted representations elicit projections toward the patient: namely, this is not psychoanalysis—leave this to medical professionals. Instead, the analyst can call on familiar interventions that are just as therapeutic even when the starkness of bodily states confuses us. First, the analyst modulates between somatic regulation and the world of the imagination competing for the patient from the thrall of the sensate, the pull of the autistic, with gestures that preserve relatedness. Second, we hold in trust a sense of the future even in the face of experiences that represent a negation of life (Harvey Peskin, personal communication, 1995). Finally, by telling stories from the countertransference, we provide language imagining aloud new possibilities.

I conclude with a story that sharply contrasts with the opening story from the analytic meetings. This one came from the *New York Times*. It was about a new medical technique that was being tried on a fire captain who had been badly burned. The treatment involved partial anesthesia with a morphine derivative to keep the patient conscious, yet at some distance from the excruciating pain, in hopes that by muting the physiological pain response healing could be facilitated. The reporter described the room with its panoply of doctors, nurses and equipment. In passing, the story mentioned that, in the midst of this scene, the captain's wife sat at his bedside holding his hand and softly singing "You Are My Sunshine". As I read this story, I thought about the sensation of her hand on his, the tone of her voice as providing her physically and psychologically traumatized husband with secure holding at the level of the autistic-contiguous position. On this man's behalf, I felt pleased and relieved to read that one therapist had been allowed in the room.

References

Cohen, J. (1985). Trauma and repression. *Psychoanalytic Inquiry*, 5: 163–189.

Feigelson, C. (1993). Personality death, object loss and the uncanny. *International Journal of Psychoanalysis*, 74: 331–345.

Gaddini, R. (1987). Early care and the roots of internalization. *International Review of Psychoanalysis*, 14: 321–332.

Hall, D. (1966). *The Old Life*. New York: Houghton Mifflin.

Khan, M. (1972). Dread of surrender to resourceless dependence. *International Journal of Psychoanalysis*, 53: 225–230.

Kinston, W. & Cohen, J. (1986). Primal repression: Clinical and theoretical aspects. *International Journal of Psychoanalysis*, 67: 337–355.

Kirshner, L.A. (1994). Trauma, the good object, and the symbolic: A theoretical integration. *International Journal of Psychoanalysis*, 75(2): 235–242.

Krystal, H. (1985). Trauma and the stimulus barrier. *Psychoanalytic Inquiry*, 5: 131–161.

Laub, D. & Auerhahn, N. (1993). Knowing and not knowing massive psychic: Forms of psychic memory. *International Journal of Psychoanalysis*, 74: 287–302.

Mayer, E. (1994). Some implications for psychoanalytic technique drawn from analysis of a dying patient. *Psychoanalytic Quarterly*, 63: 1–19.
Ogden, T. (1991a). Analyzing the matrix of transference. *International Journal of Psychoanalysis*, 72: 593–605.
Ogden, T. (1991b). Some theoretical considerations on personal isolation: A breakdown of subjectivity and intersubjectivity. *Psychoanalytic Dialogues*, 1: 377–390.
Winnicott, D.W. (1969). The use of the object. *International Journal of Psychoanalysis*, 50: 711–716.

Chapter 6

The Icarus complex and the trauma of falling forever

W. Preston Lear

> It's suicide without the commitment.
>
> Joe Weber (BASE jumper, 2007)

Much has been written about the holding function of the environmental mother. When the child suffers an inordinate lack of this provision, he can be overwhelmed by a feeling of falling forever (Winnicott, 1960/1965).[1] An omnipotent response to this psychic trauma can take the form of intense physical enactment, sometimes in sports. Activities such as rock climbing, big mountain free skiing and BASE jumping are commonly referred to as *extreme*, or action sports. When these motivated athletes pursue their dangerous games, they leave the more risk averse among us bewildered. "Because it's there" was George Mallory's retort when asked of his ambition to be the first to summit Mount Everest—enigmatic rhetoric when we consider his bold and ultimately fatal endeavor (New York Times, 1923, p. 1).

Research on the risk-taking athlete has typically been the domain of social psychologists (Johnsgard, 1968; Zuckerman, 1979; Farley, 1986). Their findings show that this class of athlete has an unusually high capacity for arousal, and exhibits features of narcissism, extroversion and creativity. Lacking in this line of research is an appreciation for unconscious motivation: how the strivings of the extreme athlete anesthetizes him from the psychic pain of having been dropped. In this chapter I add a psychoanalytic perspective to the subject, and I wish to identify how this athlete's extreme enactment is a response to early trauma. I formulate my thesis in terms of an Icarus complex.

In Ovid's version of the classic myth, Icarus and his father, Daedalus, are exiled to the outer reaches of Crete for the father's offense to King Minos. Daedalus is a master craftsman, and he fashions wings of wax and feathers in hopes of deliverance. Anticipating the exuberance of his son, Daedalus warns Icarus to fly neither too low nor too high, as the heat of the sun would melt the wax and the mist of the sea would drench the feathers. The two practice flying and, when they are confident in their abilities, resolve to escape. During the fateful flight Icarus ignores his father's directives and flies boldly toward the sun. Daedalus lacks the strength of youth to fly after Icarus, and he can only watch helplessly as his son eventually plummets to his death.

The Icarus myth contains themes of hubris and failed ambition. I believe this timeless narrative illuminates the omnipotent strivings of the patient who is enlivened from being dropped. Henry Murray (1938/2008), a psychoanalyst and personality psychologist, originally conceived of an Icarus complex, emphasizing a personality pattern containing narcissistic features that defended against a fear of failure—a neurotic-level conflict. Murray (1955/1981) also refers to this complex as a "theory of insupport," giving a nod to the enduring impact of early trauma. What Murray lacked was the expanded understanding of narcissism, put forth by his contemporaries across the pond. As object relations theory privileges the earliest experiences of relational attachment, it also serves to illuminate the primitive underpinnings of the "Icarian". Drawing from object relations theory and more recent psychoanalytic contributions, I propose an augmented formulation of an Icarus complex—an enlivened solution rooted in the infant's cumulative trauma (Khan, 1963).

Winnicott (1971), in his introduction to his paper on play, writes: "I am trying to explore an idea that has been forced on me by my work, and also forced on me by my own stage of development at the present time, which gives my work a certain colouring" (p. 51). Indeed, the ideas of an Icarus complex have been forced on me by my own work—and my own play. I am no stranger to sports of risk, and I have forged friendships with accomplished athletes—some of whom have perished in the dangerous game. Thus, my intimacy with the subject gives my thesis a "certain colouring". The majority of my days are now spent in the comparative safety of the consulting room. However, experiences with certain patients have further refined my thinking, giving my ideas of an Icarus complex a developed pair of wings, metaphorically speaking.

In the first part of this chapter I describe the prominent features of an Icarus complex. Just as the extreme athlete served as my muse, he will also provide an illustrative backdrop for my thesis. BASE jumping is a highly technical activity that involves leaping with a canopy (a parachute) from a fixed object rather than skydiving from an airplane. BASE is an acronym of the different mediums from which these athletes leap: buildings, antennas, spans (bridges) and earth (cliffs). With a heightened risk of injury or death as criteria, "BASE", as referred to by its adherents, could be considered the most extreme of action sports (Earl, 2009). As BASE athletes artfully play with flight, their calculated plunge is suggestive of Icarus; but, rather than fighting against gravity, they are embracing it with hopes of mastering its pull with a successful landing. The inherent risk of this sport is indicated by its mortality rate: an average of one death for every 2400 jumps (Di Giovanni, 2004).

An understanding of how early trauma manifests in an Icarus complex allows for a nuanced view of a BASE athlete, and a more dynamic perspective views the athlete's performance as adaptive and creative rather than merely a reckless stunt. The infant's subjective experience of falling forever is experienced in the psyche and the soma. Reenacting this trauma, deliberately engaging in dangerous pursuits, is a *feeling toned* activity (Jung, 1960), and it is an unconscious effort to master early environmental failure. Recognizing this response to trauma, while appreciating the mutable nature and dialectic tension that takes place within the complex, informs the analyst who attempts to hold this flighty individual.

In the final part of the chapter, I discuss how aspects of early trauma are inevitably enacted in the treatment relationship. Predictably, the hazardous displays of the Icarian are prone to provoke countertransference reactions that, much like a failed parachute, collapse an analytic attitude. Rather than being inducted into a possible sadomasochistic enactment, the analyst can use the patient's creatively provocative material to provide a holding environment. Here I draw from clinical examples to illustrate the challenges and risks when working with this population. A successful treatment will not entirely replace the "rush" sought after by the Icarian, just as it cannot remove the scars from archaic injury. Ultimately, the Icarian's experience of a *secure* base may liberate him from the psychic exile that compels his addictive activity, and he may be more available for the adventures that come with relational contact.

The Icarus complex

Through his extreme activity, the Icarian endeavors to gain mastery over a crushing feeling of deadness. In this portion of the chapter I present the features of an Icarus complex, all of which combine in turning a passive experience into an enlivening enactment. Some features, such as manic defense and omnipotence, emerge early in the infant's development. Oedipal conflict and exhibitionism manifest in later stages of object relating. But I emphasize that the ontogeny of these elements is rooted in early psychic injury.

Manic defense and omnipotence

According to Melanie Klein (1935/1986) a caregiver's lack of attunement leaves the child feeling dropped, and the child resorts to mania to defend against the depressive anxieties of object dependence. She argues that with omnipotence, the child "endeavors ceaselessly to *master and control* its objects, and the evidence of this effort is its hyperactivity" (p. 133). Extreme sports are disciplined distractions that bolster the Icarian's sense of invulnerability. The athletes often refer to a "rush" that is wedded to their compulsive activity. This rush, this "exaggerated liveliness" (Winnicott, 1954–5/1958, p. 272a) sought out by the extreme athlete, diminishes the feelings of deadness that consume the psyche-soma.

The somatosensory Holy Grail associated with these risky disciplines has inspired the lay diagnosis of "adrenaline junkie"—a label as pejorative as it is reductionistic. Max Knutson (2009), an active BASE jumper, counters:

> People assume that we're adrenaline junkies. We're not. The reason I jump is because when I'm standing on the edge my head is clearer than anything. It doesn't matter that you got a speeding ticket, or you lost your job. Just pure clarity, better than meditation. Few people are in control of their lives, and when you're falling at 180 miles-per-hour and you've got the ability and knowledge to survive that, that's control. The power of controlling your fears is insurmountable. (p. 3)

A corollary of this activity is an unconscious wish to destroy the object—there will be others long burdened with the consequences of the BASE jumper's fatal leap. His obliterating the internalized bad object involves his projection of need. If we expand from a Kleinian notion of omnipotence to a paradigm of interrelatedness, the addictive rush sought by the Icarian is over-determined. Let us assume that the infant who feels dropped has had some experience of being held. Subsequent to injury, the sensitive child may experience the object mother as unavailable to be used by the infant, since the environment mother has dropped the infant and is reified into a version that is all bad (Winnicott, 1962/1965). The Icarian's manic activity is a regressive attempt to merge with an idealized version of the internal relationship. This regressive attempt at fusion with the "almighty mother" is the heir to narcissistic object-relating (Chasseguet-Smirgel, 1984). Michael Diamond (2014) explains: "Some children trapped in their own disproportionate narcissism get caught in a self-destructive upwards spiral of manic activity, flying higher to avoid facing the panic of being unable to rejoin the object from which they have tried to separate."

Climb and fall

In *Thrills and Regressions* Michael Balint (1959) writes of two manifestations for the child who suffers a rupture in his holding environment. I draw heavily from one of them, the *philobat*, in addressing the Icarian's inclination to climb and fall. Balint's philobat is one who enjoys thrills involving "high speed, exposed situations, and completely new forms of satisfaction" (p. 25). In contrast to the ocnophile, "one who prefers to clutch at something firm when his security is in danger" (p. 25), the philobat's observable behaviors manifest the opposite inclination—he prefers to push away from the object, "proving [his] independence … when away from safety" (p. 28). It is as if the BASE jumper and other extreme athletes served as models for Balint's observations. After ascending the medium from which he will jump—an ascent that is often technical and dangerous itself—the athlete deliberately falls of his own accord. His skillful exploits engender a sense of mastery, but this reenactment does little to foster relational contact. Balint elaborates: "Although in their deeper layer philobatic thrills represent the primal scene, phenomenologically they are much nearer to autoeroticism. Philobatic heroism is, in a way, phallic-narcissistic heroism, most manly and at the same time very childish, never fully mature" (p. 44).

I recall seeing a rock climber donning a t-shirt that read: "Climbing may be hard, but it's easier than growing up." A degree of obsessive narcissism is required to engage at a high level in most any activity; the athlete must, as Balint put it, "submit his performance to incessant, exacting reality testing, and to searching self-criticism" (p. 84). For the extreme athlete this reality testing occurs within the treacherous playing field, both a literal and radical *environment mother* that consists of steep rock walls, big waves or precarious edges—all features of an object less threatening than (and reminiscent of) the internalized source of the original trauma (Winnicott, 1962/1965). Christopher Bollas (1979) lends harmony with his concept, *aesthetic of being*, which emerges when an early breach of the infant–mother relationship motivates a transformational reenactment. The extreme athlete—whether he is a climber, a skier or a BASE jumper—will refer to the "committing lines" in reverential tones. These specific lines, the course of the athlete's ascent/descent, are framed by the contours of mother earth. Surviving the dance in this breathtaking environment sustains the jouissance associated with his sport. And it is in this awe-inspiring playground that the athlete maintains an idealized connection with an ethereal object.

Exhibitionism

Prompted by the sun's central role in the Icarus narrative, Murray (1955/1981) coined the feature *cynosural* narcissism: "This strikes me as a suitable term (more embracing than exhibitionism) to denote a craving for unsolicited attention and admiration, a desire to attract and enchant all eyes, like a star in the firmament" (p. 549). Considering the thrill-seeking athlete, I believe phallic-narcissism—an exhibitionistic phallic-narcissism—is more encompassing than Murray's term. Just like the other features of an Icarus complex, this exhibition is rooted in an early rupture. The infant who is falling forever does not feel held by his mother's gaze.

Short of the canopy, no piece of equipment receives more attention from the BASE athlete than the camera (Weber, 2007). Some jumpers employ multiple cameras, and energy spent on filming blurs the line between sport and performance art. Point-of-view (POV) cameras adorn many an athlete's helmet and allow him to post his adventures immediately online (Kronick, 2013). Athletes acknowledge that "Kodak courage" can be a compelling motivator, and capturing images allows the aesthetic moment a longer shelf life. Smart phones store footage, and *action selfies* allow the athlete to both scrutinize and cling to the experience. The added element of performing to be seen can also present a hazardous distraction to an activity that requires focus of the participant. Tragically, a recent BASE fatality was attributed to a young woman's canopy wrapping around the mount of her helmet camera (Di Giovanni, 2010).

Oedipal conflict

I have emphasized that the Icarian's compulsive activity has an archaic foundation that pre-dates the oedipal drama, and it involves, in part, an unconscious wish to merge with the idealized mother. But in the Icarus complex we also observe features of competitive striving, castration anxiety and defiance: hallmark features of oedipal conflict (Freud, 1900).

Legal strictures limiting the activity of BASE contribute to an inherent, anti-authoritarianism in the sport. In 1999 Frank Gambalie, a prolific BASE athlete, brazenly jumped Yosemite National Park's Half Dome at midday. To evade park officials intent on arresting him, Gambalie dived into the rapids of the Merced River and drowned while still in his harness. On the heels of Gambalie's death, a protest jump involving five athletes was organized from Yosemite's El Capitan with intent to defy authorities and to demonstrate that BASE jumping within national parks could be accomplished safely. During this publicized event, Jan Davis failed to deploy her canopy. Assuming her equipment would be confiscated, Davis used borrowed gear that had been rigged for a left-handed jumper. She was unable to reach the ripcord (Gutman and Fredrick, 2002). What are we to make of this tragic irony? Was her defiance so consuming that it ushered in a hysterical lapse in view of the paternal order?

Many traditions contain a narrative of a father's sins being visited on the heads of his sons. Preceding the patricide in Sophocles' *Oedipus Rex* is the murderous intent of Oedipus' father, Laius (Le Guen, 1974). Early in the story, Laius, fearing for his own life, orders his infant son to be put to death. Indeed, it is Laius' folly of defying the gods that sets in motion a transgenerational pattern of violence and trauma. Returning to the Icarus myth, Daedalus' "sins of the father" set the stage. It is noteworthy that there is no mention of Icarus' mother or of Daedalus' wife. According to ancient writers, Icarus was the son of Naucrate, a 15-year-old Minoan slave-girl of King Minos. Years later, an envious Daedalus murders his talented nephew, Talos, a crime that was a harbinger of later crimes against the King. Given the competitive striving that later unfolds, perhaps fate would not allow the violent uncle to succeed as a compassionate father. As the master craftsman formulates a means of escape, Daedalus is mindful of the risks of flight, and he warns Icarus to fly a middle course. The youth's lofty flight is a revolt against his aging father, and suggests Icarus' identification with a more powerful father-sun-god. In other traditions we observe how devotion (ambition?) engenders acts of sacrificial, masochistic and murderous intent; and this range of enactments influence a parallel development between father and child: there is Abraham, who is stopped just short of killing his son, Isaac; and Jesus, beseeching his heavenly father from the cross. Jesus' questioning God for forsaking him reflected both his separate identity from the father and his realization of humanity. Likewise, Icarus' omnipotence is shattered when his fashioned wings fail. His realization of the paternal universe, one that he does not control, is manifest as he falls headlong into mother-ocean (*La Mer*).

Creativity

Charles Brenner (1982) expresses a view of the extreme athlete that, while not altogether misinformed, is limited: "being counterphobic by becoming a daredevil and delighting in doing what is realistically dangerous is a symptom" (p. 90). I implore that the grounded participant allow for an attitude that is more analytic and less pathologizing. If we appreciate the athlete's activity as a form of artistic expression, we can interpret his quest for mastery as both destructive *and* potentially creative.

As the Icarian's art takes place in a deadly medium, at what point does his creative performance give way to a counterphobic enactment with catastrophic results? In "The Vital Role of Adaptive Grandiosity in Artistic Creativity", Peter Wolson (1995) addresses the precarious balance that fuels artistic enterprise. Applying his ideas to the endeavors of the Icarian offers an enriched perspective for the extreme athlete. Wolson describes adaptive grandiosity as predominantly a manic defense, and he argues that it is the artist's "exhilarating conviction of his potential for greatness" that compels not only his single-minded effort to cultivate his craft but also to display "the content of his inner world through his creative medium" (p. 578). This proclivity only becomes maladaptive when it reaches a level of omnipotence, thereby impeding independent creativity and learning from experience. Icarus, adorned with Daedalus' wings, displays a flight toward the heavens. His lofty course displays his own signature, extending the limits of his father's creation. The most impressive rock climbs demand a creative vision from the climber. First ascents require a base of knowledge to be applied to the untouched medium. The BASE athlete will often seek out a first *descent*—a "creative line" that has never been jumped. This feat is revered if it is accomplished with flair and "good style": How close to the cliff face was the athlete able to track? How long did he delay before pulling open his canopy?

Experienced extreme athletes develop the capacity to turn back on jumps or ski runs that, after assessing all the variables, may be too dangerous at the moment. "Live to ski another day" was a friend's refrain when he and I backed away from skiing our intended steep and untracked slope—a destination that demanded a five-hour climb. Assessing all the variables, some of which could not have been accurate unless we were atop the slope itself, yielded sufficient signs of avalanche risk. These *objective hazards*, as they are called in avalanche safety parlance, were enough to sway our subjective decision. If the unfortunate Icarus had tempered his ambitions he might have struck a balance: his strength allowing him to fly to greater heights than his father; and the increased altitude providing space for an artful, exhilarating and survivable descent.

Clinical example: Sharon

Twenty-five years ago Sharon shelved her aspirations to be a world-class mountain climber for a more traditional path of marriage and motherhood. She arrived at my office having survived a string of suicide attempts and hospitalizations. I found my eyes drawn to the scars from knee-replacement surgeries, scars that offered lasting evidence of the lengths to which she continues to push herself physically. Now in her fifties, Sharon spends more time on the golf course than in the mountains; but her destructive enactments are more overt than that of most extreme athletes in their prime.

Sharon's initial suicide attempt immediately followed the death of her mother. This violent act was followed by more loss: Her father died suddenly of a heart attack; and her husband of 25 years, the father of their three children, filed for divorce. This confluence of trauma ushered in a pattern more of suicide attempts and hospitalizations for the next five years. The fact that she survived her most recent overdose of pills and alcohol left physicians baffled and Sharon frustrated. While in the hospital, Sharon divulged that she had been raped repeatedly by her ex-husband over the last half of their marriage—a shameful secret that served to amplify her sense of isolation and failure, for she had been raised in a family where vulnerability was inadmissible and daughter-wife-mother were expected to be "perpetually positive".

Opportunities afforded by her family's affluence did not compensate for Sharon's emotional impoverishment. Her parents lacked the capacity to allow for a range of feelings in their sensitive child, and the shadow of the *object* fell upon Sharon. The lion's share of her inheritance was a haunting sense of inadequacy, emptiness and shame.

When she was a girl in grade school Sharon broke her arm in the playground. Her mother initially doubted the validity of the x-rays, and was furious with Sharon for requiring a cast for her arm. Upon hearing this traumatic account, I was struck by the distance from her feelings of rage and grief toward her mother. When asked about her thoughts of this painful memory, her answer hearkened to Nietzsche's (1888/1990) maxim on that which does not kill us. She offered: "I guess it toughened me up to overcome my later injuries."

The athletic arena provided a sanctioned venue for Sharon's aggression. Her initial attempt at differentiation from her parents involved her giving up a track and field scholarship for the demanding activity of high-altitude mountaineering. Tragedy struck when two in her all-women party perished in an avalanche in the Andes. Sharon explained that her survivor's guilt was amplified by the sexist diatribes that followed, such as, "Women are simply less equipped to function at high altitude." Even though Sharon had not made an overtly bad call on the mountain, the harsh criticism from some in the climbing community deepened her wounds. Shortly afterward Sharon left her beloved mountains and returned to university. She married two years later.

From the outset of our working together, Sharon's buzzing agitation and maniacal determination to "make progress every session" defended her from feelings of deadness. During the painstaking process in which she shared more horrors perpetuated at the hands of her now ex-husband, I began to recognize the backdrop of early trauma. It was in moments when she felt most alone, those corresponding with weekends and other ruptures in treatment, that Sharon often retreated to the "rush" made possible by a bottle of chardonnay with a handful of Klonopin as chaser. Working with Sharon was a course in curbing my therapeutic ambition. My own analysis and supervision made possible a capacity to make meaning of her provocative and masochistic attacks.

Now, a few years later, things have begun to shift for Sharon. She can still feel like a hot potato, but is more able to allow me to "be alone in the room with [her]" (Bolgar, 2012). Sharon is more able to talk—and think—about her enlivening flights. A year following her last suicide attempt she commenced training as a volunteer for a suicide hotline. Sharon acknowledges this is an evocative choice for a volunteer job, and her identification with callers provides material for her own treatment. In a recent session, Sharon displayed the features of her Icarus complex, demonstrating how the manifestations of cumulative trauma fuel her enlivening pursuits:

> I just love this work, Dr. Lear. I love the intensity. I love the adrenaline that comes with helping people when they are in crisis. I think it's the reality of death and what could happen that I find so exciting and so … alive.

In a recent session with Sharon my thoughts returned to Nietzsche (1886/1997): "we are in the midst of our bliss only when we are the most in danger." Sharon explained:

> These adrenalizing situations … even the feeling I get after, when I've determined to take a handful of pills … I guess it's that … it's a feeling. I've always been drawn to intensity. You know that, like intense sports. But when everything happened five years ago, when I was so alone, I didn't have any feeling at all. And that's more dreadful than anything.

Later we talked about my upcoming vacation, and Sharon speculated as to where I might go. (Early in our work together she had noticed surfboards atop my car, and she correctly assumed that this trip would involve waves and warm water.) Sharon then associated to the prospective victims of a looming hurricane off the coast of Mexico: "I really feel sorry for so many of the people who live in its path, whose houses are less secure … whose houses don't have a secure foundation. They're really that much more … more exposed when the storm hits."

My mind went to the storms of abuse and betrayal that Sharon has suffered as an adult, and her ongoing struggles to withstand the unpredictable gusts of post-traumatic stress. I believe that Sharon was also alluding to the fallout from basic fault of having been dropped—a rupture that was reinvigorated following her mother's death.

Near-death in the consulting room

Aspects of a trauma history inevitably emerge in enactments within the treatment relationship. For the extreme athlete, the reality of physical injury is the price of admission for the privileged ride. Hence, the Icarian's violence toward the soma is not secretive. As he hobbles into the office on crutches, he broadcasts both his pain and his aggression. The analyst will witness painful recoveries following the patient's myriad accidents during a course of treatment. Indeed, the single-minded intention of the athlete recovering from his physical injury, and his omnipotent resolve to rise from the ashes to fly again, highlight the overdetermined relationship with his sport.

In "Addiction to Near-Death", Betty Joseph (1982) writes of the patient who is so intent on self-destruction that his sadomasochistic enactments dominate all aspects of his life. She describes the person in the throes of this addiction as "withdraw[ing] into a secret world of violence that … is often physically expressed" (p. 10). I believe Joseph's assertion applies to the Icarian: "Indeed, in all these patients the place where the pull towards near-death is most obvious is in the transference" (p. 1).

Indeed, this injury–recovery pattern suggests the sadomasochistic bond to a rejecting/dropping object (Fairbairn, 1944). But Joseph makes clear that the patient's powerful masochism pulls for a collusion of despair in which the analyst becomes harsh or critical in some way toward the patient: "then both patient and analyst go down in failure" (1982, p. 20). Again, the Icarian has been dropped, and this time he has orchestrated the fall in the transference–countertransference relationship.

The analyst is most effective as he develops a balance between supporting the impassioned pursuit of the Icarian while not colluding with the patient's defenses. An analytic attitude in the face of such destructive forces calls for what Stephen Mitchell (1986) refers to as a *synthetic approach* involving "both a playful participation in the patient's illusions and a puzzled curiosity about how and why [these enactments] came to be the sine qua non of the analysand's sense of security and involvements with others" (p. 125).

Clinical example: Paul

Paul is a multi-talented man in his early thirties who struggled in his career as a mechanical engineer. His narrative included unrealized potential as an artist and athlete, and he felt the responsibilities of marriage and fatherhood to be persecuting limitations, similar to a crippling knee injury that cut short his ambitions for ski racing.

Paul came to my office on the recommendation from one of his friends at the gym. Within the first minute of our meeting, Paul wasted no time in presenting challenges to come:

> I understand that you're a clinician who is training to become a psychoanalyst. If you were to take me on as, what is it called, a "control case?" ... it might provide me an affordable opportunity to learn about psychoanalysis. And, since you're in training, perhaps you might be able to learn from me as well.

It did not take long for the effects of Paul's early trauma, that of having been dropped, to play out in the transference–countertransference relationship. Cumulative injury from a borderline mother and later slights from a rejecting father informed Paul's relational life. Indeed, my patient's prophecy of my learning from him came to fruition, for it demanded more than I alone could muster to withstand his barrage of anal-sadistic attacks.

Paul often led sessions by describing persistent physical injuries suffered from martial arts or intense workouts at the gym. Early in the treatment I heard these accounts as repetition of his early trauma—passive psychic injury was turned into active harm to the soma. My thoughts also went to Freud's reference to the tooth-ache and narcissistic withdrawal: "a person who is tormented by organic pain and discomfort gives up his interest in the things of the external world, in so far as they do not concern his suffering" (1914, p. 82). With time I experienced Paul's frequent physical injuries, along with the accompanying perseveration, as a challenging barrier to relational contact.

The following statement is an example of Paul's flighty ideations: "My daughter was playing like she was Tinker Bell, and we both fantasized about fairy dust. Oh, how I wish I had fairy dust! Then I could fly around all the time and not have to worry about it." In turn, I found that I was left worrying about Paul's (Peter Pan's?) participation in activities that are usually the domain of youth in their teens and twenties. However, I did not recognize Paul's physical features that suggested an Icarus complex until he arrived at my office with stitches across his forehead. Paul's parents were visiting from out of town, and, as his family watched from the porch, he failed to land a rather technical trick with his skateboard.

One of Paul's hobbies involved refurbishing Vespa scooters. He spoke fondly of buzzing through stop-and-go traffic on his latest restoration. I recall thinking it was a good thing that Paul was savvy with a wrench: He was in three accidents in his first year of treatment—two of them en route to my office. During sessions he relayed many more near misses at the hands of "stupid California drivers". As a former bicycle commuter, I was familiar with my fellow citizens' practice of driving sport-utility vehicles while texting. One morning, after Paul related an accident that had totaled his Vespa and luckily left him with nary a scratch, I gently commented: "The roads around here are perilous on a scooter, especially given the distracted drivers over whom you have no control."

Paul's rejoinder conveyed his level of persecution: "I have been riding Vespas my entire life! And I'm safe! It's the stupid drivers' fault! And I'm not about to just sit on my ass in traffic in a big, old car." Later we were able to explore how Paul felt attacked. He had experienced me as a harsh and ignorant authority—one who drives an old car and aims to clip his wings.

In the months that followed, Paul developed some capacity to recognize the limits of his omnipotence. Paul no longer arrived to session with his helmet under his arm. He reserved his Vespa adventures to rides within his neighborhood. The terrain of treatment began to deepen to the psychic injuries of his having felt dropped by his parents. He was even able to voice how terrifying it was for him to depend on me.

At 22 months into his analysis, Paul suddenly announced his intention to "take a break". He explained that he needed to focus more on developing his career, and that he planned to return to analysis when he had more time and money. I reminded Paul that he had previously expressed concerns that I was going to "drop" him when we reached the two-year mark of his analysis (unfortunately he had learned of the time requirement for training cases at my institute). I also interpreted that the timing of his retreat may be a pre-emptive strike. Paul would hear none of this, and I was left with a feeling of helpless and persecuted rage: It was tragic that he was retreating at a moment when his analysis was on the cusp of relational contact! It was not lost on me that his retreat was also a sadistic victory that adversely affected my own career development, at least in terms of my completing a two-year training case.

Betty Joseph (1982) emphasizes that "in the transference one gets the feeling of being driven up to the edge of things … both the patient and the analyst feel tortured" (p. 10). An Icarus complex involves expensive thrills, both for the Icarian and those who attempt to join him.

Clinical example: Sharon

I would now like to revisit Sharon, the woman in my practice whom I mentioned earlier. You will recall the session in which we discussed her penchant for "feeling adrenalized". Toward the end of the hour Sharon talked about her having let her pilot's license lapse: "I just don't need the temptation. Besides, I've kind of lost interest because the only exciting part involved the take-off and landing." I commented that with her being enamored with, even enlivened by, the prospect of death, there were also parts of her that wished to continue living.

Patients who spurn their feelings of need *doth protest too much.* The Icarian's negation of need displays his longing to be held (Freud, 1925). Sharon ended the session with a ray of hope:

> Well, I guess it involves a letting go, less of a fight … like when I was whitewater kayaking in the Kern [River]. I remember getting flipped upside down during a crucial stretch of rapids. I freaked out, and then I was able to loosen and quit fighting in such a gripped way. I then released from out of my kayak, and the river's current pushed me into a huge eddy. It was still scary, but I was out of the more dangerous part of the run. [Laughs] But then again, I would have stayed there, stuck in the eddy, had someone not come by and helped me out.

Conclusion

The risk-taker's compulsion can leave the analyst feeling as helpless as Daedalus, who could do little more than witness his son's perilous course. Insisting that the Icarian relinquish his wings is an omnipotent (more accurately, *impotent*) directive. But the therapist can carry hope, a hope that the analytic adventure may open additional avenues for this driven individual. Over what will likely be a long, bumpy flight for both members of the thinking couple, the Icarian may loosen his grip on an idealized attachment and be freed to experience a deeper joy in his creative activity. Emboldened from the holding experience, this patient may begin to take the greatest risk of all: loving outside of himself.

Note

1 An earlier version of this chapter won the Michael J. Diamond Candidate Essay Award in 2014 given by the Los Angeles Institute and Society for Psychoanalytic Studies (LAISPS).

References

Balint, M. (1959). *Thrills and Regressions.* New York: International Universities Press.

Bolgar, H. (2012). Personal conversation. Los Angeles, California.

Bollas, C. (1979). The transformational object. *International Journal of Psychoanalysis*, 60: 97–107.

Brenner, C. (1982). *The Mind in Conflict.* Madison: International Universities Press.

Chasseguet-Smirgel, J. (1984). *Creativity and Perversion.* New York: Norton.

Di Giovanni, N. (2004). BASE jumping history. *Basic Research.* Retrieved June 3, 2005, from http://www.basicresearch.com/base_history.htm.

Di Giovanni, N. (2010). BASE fatality list. Retrieved July 10, 2010, from http://www.splatula.com/bfl.

Diamond, M. (2014). Discussion of W. Preston Lear's "The Icarus Complex and the Addiction to Near-Death". Presented at LAISPS scientific meeting. Los Angeles, California.

Earl, J. (2009). *Extreme Sports.* Broomwall, PA: Mason Crest.

Fairbairn, R. (1944). Endopsychic structure considered in terms of object relationships. *International Journal of Psychoanalysis*, 25: 70–92.

Farley, F. (1986). The big T personality. *Psychology Today*, 20: 45–52.

Freud, S. (1900a). The interpretation of dreams. *Standard Edition 4–5*: 1–626. London: Hogarth Press.

Freud, S. (1914b). On narcissism: An introduction. *Standard Edition 14*: 67–102. London: Hogarth Press.

Freud, S. (1925). Negation. *Standard Edition 19*: 235–239. London: Hogarth Press.

Gutman, B. & Frederick, S. (2002). *Being Extreme: Thrills and Dangers in the World of Extreme Sports.* New York: Kensington.

Johnsgard, K. (1968). The competitive racing driver: A preliminary report. *Journal of Sports Medicine and Physical Fitness*, 15(2): 87–95.

Joseph, B. (1982). Addiction to near-death. *International Journal of Psychoanalysis*, 63: 449–456.

Jung, C.G. (1960). *On the Nature of the Psyche.* Translated by R.F.C. Hull. Princeton, NJ: Princeton University Press.

Khan, M. (1963). The concept of cumulative trauma. *Psychoanalytic Study of the Child*, 18: 286–306.

Klein, M. (1935/1986). A contribution to the psychogenisis of manic-depressive states. *The Selected Melanie Klein*, J. Mitchell (ed.). New York: The Free Press.

Knutson, M. (2009). Blinc forum. *Blinc Magazine.* Retrieved August 12, 2009 from http://www.blincmagazine.com/forum/original-base-board/4262-mick-knutson.

Kronick, J. (2013). *The World of Red Bull.* Documentary segment on *Real Sports*, HBO.

Le Guen, C. (1974). The formation of transference: On the Laius complex in the armchair. *International Journal of Psychoanalysis*, 55: 505–512.

Mitchell, S. (1986). The wings of Icarus. *Contemporary Psychoanalysis*, 22: 107–132.

Murray, H. (1938/2008). *Explorations in Personality.* New York: Oxford University Press.

Murray, H. (1955/1981). American Icarus. *Clinical Studies of Personality*, A. Burton & R. Harris (eds.). New York: Harper & Row, 615–641.

Nietzsche, F. (1886/1997). *Beyond Good and Evil.* Mineola, NY: Dover Publications.

Neitzsche, F. (1888/1990) *Twilight of the Idols and the Anti-Christ, or How to Philosophize with a Hammer.* London: Penguin.

New York Times. (1923, March 18). Climbing Mount Everest is work for supermen.

Weber, J. (2007). BASEwiki. *Blinc Magazine.* Blincmagazine.com.

Winnicott, D.W. (1954–5/1958). The depressive position in normal emotional development. *Collected Papers.* New York: Basic Books.

Winnicott, D.W. (1960/1965). Ego distortion in terms of true and false self. *Maturational Processes and the Facilitating Environment: Studies in the Theory of Emotional Development.* New York: International Universities Press, 140–152.

Winnicott, D.W. (1962/1965). Ego integration in child development. *The Maturational Processes and the Facilitating Environment: Studies in the Theory of Emotional Development.* New York: International Universities Press, 56–63.

Winnicott, D.W. (1971). *Playing and Reality.* London: Penguin.
Wolson, P. (1995). The vital role of adaptive grandiosity in artistic creativity. *Psychoanalytic Review,* 82: 577–597.
Zuckerman, M. (1979). *Sensation Seeking: Beyond the Optimal Level of Arousal.* Hillsdale, NJ: Erlbaum.

Chapter 7

Psychic deadness and the vicissitudes of unmetabolized mourning

Maxine Nelson

> I've seen things you people wouldn't believe. Attack ships on fire off the shoulder of Orion. I've watched C-beams glitter in the dark near the Tannhauser Gate. All those moments will be lost in time, like tears in rain. Time to die.
>
> Roy Batty soliloquy, *Blade Runner* (1982/2007)

In this chapter I will explore the experience of psychic deadness in the long-term treatment of a middle-aged man with significant psychotic features. The material I will discuss is predominantly clinical, although I will also discuss some theoretical concepts that have proved invaluable in my understanding of, and work with, this patient.

Blade Runner: an organizing metaphor

In the second week of a four-times-weekly treatment that is currently in its fourteenth year, I invited Sam, then 30, to tell me a bit about his mother. As if he had anticipated my question, Sam made an association to the opening scene of *Blade Runner*, in which Leon Kowalski, a suspected replicant (that is, a genetically engineered human with a four-year lifespan), shoots dead the investigator who has asked him to talk about *his* mother. While I was initially puzzled by this association, over time I came to understand it both as a warning to me not to probe any deeper, and as a sign of Sam's frustration and fear of being exposed to me as less than human.

Leon's rage in the film—mirroring my patient's rage and despair about his life—is related to the fact that replicants don't have mothers, a condition that identifies them as not fully human and therefore subject to killing if they are found in areas forbidden (by their human creators) to their kind. Their motherlessness leaves them vulnerable in two other ways as well: in the feeling that they are "different"; and, more specifically, in the fact that they have never learned to navigate painful emotions, both in themselves and in relation to others. Although Sam did, of course, have an actual mother, he, like the replicants, lacked the inner experience of a maternal object sturdy enough to contain both his loving impulses and his destructive ones. Without sufficient containing function within the mother–infant dyad, the limited capacity to hold new experience, with its inevitable pain and uncertainty, can cause infantile trauma which reverberates throughout the individual's life, inhibiting the possibility for psychic development and a sense of aliveness.

Unlike the replicant Leon, however, whose rage at his motherlessness led him to kill, I believe that Sam turned the tables of his rage—opting (unconsciously) to idealize his mother and to blame himself, both for being different from others and for failing to succeed in his life as a result. Remaining fearful of the implications of full humanity but still longing to achieve it, Sam did not end his physical life. But for many years he has trapped himself within the impoverished emotional experience that I have called "psychic deadness".

Szykierski (2010) links Bion's major contributions to psychanalytic metapsychology to his attempts at understanding the severe and long-lasting trauma he experienced as a 19-year-old tank commander in World War I. Bion called the infant's experience of having his distress signals understood and addressed *containment* (1959/1967, p. 106), and suggested that this experience is possible primarily in the context of what he called *maternal reverie* (1962/1967, p. 116)—that is, a mother's intuitive capacity to receive, understand and respond to her infant's distress by empathically lending her own mature emotional and cognitive capacities on the infant's behalf, the mother's alpha function. Her capacity to process her infant's overwhelming experience into a less toxic and more manageable form allows the child to learn to manage, and eventually integrate, progressively more challenging emotional experiences by himself. Under ideal circumstances, the infant's introjection of the mother's alpha function creates an internal space in which he can begin to build his mental structure.

When such a space is not available in his external environment, however, the distressed infant (and later child) does not feel himself safely held together. Unable to contain overwhelming mental contents by himself, he feels continually forced to evacuate them, often in the form of rage. As I will show, Sam evacuated his rage not only externally, but also into his body. Deprived of the capacity to contain rage and grief, and therefore enable successful mourning, he created a virtual life that he could retreat into and control. He created game characters whose lives he could control and run, thus functioning both as a replicant and as the genetic engineer who creates them. Unfortunately, there were psychotic dimensions to this attempt at self-protection; and over time it became a kind of autistic encapsulation that robbed him of his feelings of potency and aliveness, as well as the possibility for emotional growth.

A strong early environment of containment in the context of maternal reverie encourages the internalization of good objects and empathic processes—both of which are necessary for tolerating and dealing with painful emotional experience. Sam had few internalizations available to him as he endured a series of significant losses and traumas during latency, adolescence, and early adulthood; these were exacerbated by the suicide of the sister closest to him when he was 19.

Clinical summary

The man who I am calling Sam was referred to me in late 2005. His presenting symptoms included despair, fatigue, increased irritability with angry outbursts, and a profound sense of hopelessness. He told me in the first session that he wanted help with his pervasive feeling that "life is meaningless". Sam said that he had previously consulted with two male therapists, and expressed with some urgency that I was his "last hope". My conjecture is that his previous therapists responded to the manifest content of Sam's material, but that they did not address the more psychotic aspects, which remained hidden. My initial impression of Sam was that he was barely surviving; he was spending most of his time in bed, unmotivated even to shower and groom himself.

After graduating from college, Sam worked for a large engineering company, but he had left the workforce a number of years before we met. When I asked about this, he would mumble something about having no desire (or need) to work. He spent his time during the day playing computer games, and on weekends he played *Dungeons and Dragons* (D&D) with friends he had known since college. He had met his wife during his senior year of college, and the two of them married shortly thereafter. He described her as extremely hard working; over the years, she had risen into an upper management position for an international company. She had wanted a family, but Sam refused, fearing that his daunting family history of mental illness, about which more in a minute, might be passed on. After Sam quit his job, his wife focused most of her attention on taking care of him, essentially allowing him to become her dependent baby in perpetuity. The two of them spent their evenings together watching TV shows and movies, although she occasionally took a break from tending Sam to spend time with her family. These separations were difficult for him, as were breaks in the analysis.

Developmental history

Sam is the youngest of three children, and the only son. During his early years, his father worked as a skilled laborer, and his mother as a nurse. He explained that his parents arranged their schedules so that his father worked days and his mother worked nights. This gave Sam a sense that "someone was always there"; but, he pointed out, it also meant that someone was always absent. He had been an inquisitive child and excelled at school, particularly in math and science. Although Sam described his mother as "warm and caring", he had few recollections of receiving any help from her in understanding or managing his feelings. In his descriptions, she sounded more like what

Winnicott has called an "environmental mother" (1965, p. 47) who provided food, clothing and a stable home environment, but not the emotional holding that Winnicott considered essential to emotional and cognitive development.

In contrast to the vagueness with which he spoke about his mother, Sam emphatically described his relationship with his father as "tense and conflicted". This split was apparent in the transference, where my patient experienced me as a warm, caring maternal object when I didn't challenge him, and as a critical paternal object when I did.

Socially isolated as a child, Sam became attached to a number of pets, and told me it had been traumatic for him when they died. Although he didn't date in high school, Sam managed to find at least a few close friends, boys like himself, who were bright and highly competitive. Competition was—and still is —very important to him and he worked hard to be at the top of his class. Of his two sisters, Sam felt closest to Carrie, who was two and a half years older than him. Sam described the two of them as "being in the same orbit."

In one session at the beginning of our work together, Sam described his childhood as relatively happy. "I was taken care of by my sisters and mother," he told me, "so I didn't have to ask for anything. Maybe I was too nurtured as a kid so I got broken easily." I tried to take this comment up the next day, and was confused when he told me he had "divorced himself" from the previous material because it was painful. This would be one of the few times in Sam's long treatment where he allowed me to enter the privacy of his "internal theatre", in which experiences are able to register as emotionally painful and where previously idealized objects are able to be seen—at least briefly—in a more realistic way.

As he began to trust more in our relationship, Sam became able to talk about his conflicted relationship with his father. The young Sam felt constantly criticized and belittled by his father, as though he could never please him. Sam offered as an example the recollection (a screen memory, perhaps?) of his father kicking over the toy soldiers he liked to play with. "Crushed" by his father's repudiation of him, he ran up to his room, and cried by himself. I asked what happened after experiences like these, but Sam was vague, which led me to conjecture that Sam's mother could neither help him contain the dynamics of his relationship with his father, nor could she protect him.

Another source of tension in the family was Sam's eldest sister, Ellen, who was oppositional as a teenager and caused a great deal of anguish within the family. She married early and became psychotically depressed after her first child died of sudden infant death syndrome (SIDS) when Sam was 12. The death of his infant niece was only the beginning of the tragedies that Sam endured but was unable to suffer. His life collapsed after losing both of his sisters to suicide.

Carrie, the sister closest in age to him and the one he described as his "soul mate", was diagnosed and treated for schizophrenia in late adolescence, when she moved away to attend college. She shot and killed herself when she was 22 and Sam was 19. Two other traumatic events occurred that same year: Sam was held up at gun point, and he underwent a sexual assault from a male roommate. In both instances, Sam felt profoundly confused and alone. He was confused about his own responsibility (or not) for what had happened, and he felt no confidence that anyone, including his family, would be able to empathically receive and help him understand what it was that he had endured. I believe that the "final straw" was the death of his sister Ellen, which occurred when she was 37 and Sam 29. Ellen spent the last years of her life institutionalized, and died by asphyxiation in her car while on leave from the state hospital. Although it's unclear precisely what happened, Sam interpreted her death as a passive act of suicide. It was after Ellen's death that Sam began failing at work, which led to his eventual "retirement".

Through slow and painstaking work in his analysis, Sam was gradually able to describe how emotionally shattered he felt after Carrie's suicide. He became floridly psychotic at that time, attempting to complete his college studies while struggling with visual and auditory hallucinations, along with intense phantasies of committing suicide as part of a violent shooting spree. (This was also when he first encountered *Blade Runner*.) Sam became stabilized through his work with a female therapist at his university, and his psychotic phantasies eventually subsided (without medication) after he met his future wife during his senior year of college.

However, this was also when Sam began constructing the "psychic bunker" into which he withdrew in his efforts to survive. Time ceases to exist in the bunker, and painful or frustrating experiences are avoided at all costs. Sam's existence in the bunker consisted of spending his days playing computer games, watching hockey games (both live and taped), and engaging in various chat rooms. He went outside rarely—mostly to participate in his analysis and his weekly D&D games. He entered a twilight zone of extended melancholia at the time of Carrie's death as a means of keeping himself virtually connected with his sister, and has continued to exist within it, to a greater or lesser degree, into the present. He had married someone who reminded him of his sister, and kept her alive in his gaming by creating avatars that resemble her. Most significantly, however, he keeps himself suspended in a state where he is physically alive but psychically dead. This state, I believe, perpetuates the phantasy that time has stopped and that his sister has not died and/or that he has not killed her.

Course of treatment

Most notable to me during the first several years of Sam's treatment, when we worked face-to-face, was his manner of bombarding me with obsessive ramblings. The effusive way he gesticulated with his arms and hands reminded me of an excited infant. He also rhythmically rubbed the sides and bottoms of his feet together, intensely enough that he left tufts of wool bunched up on the area rug in front of him. My observation was that, rather than interact with me, Sam used these rhythmic movements to create a substitute reality that excluded me. In my countertransference I came to understand these movements as a kind of autistic maneuver that enabled him to be in the room with me without acknowledging that there were, in fact, two of us. Since lying on the couch, he continues to move his arms and hands in an animated way, particularly when I have said something that matches his preformed hypothesis about what is happening between us. These are moments when he feels we are in the same place—that is, occupying the same body—thus enabling him to remain fused with me and denying any object relatedness. My supposition is that since Sam's mother was unable to receive and assist him in mentalizing his emotions, he remained psychically unborn and without the experience of separateness.

The emotion that Sam was most aware of, and most comfortable with, was anger. Over time, I became aware of a history of significant verbal (and some physical) abuse toward his wife, while noticing at the same time a careful suppression of any aggressive feelings towards me in the transference. In the past, most of Sam's irritation with me had occurred when I had a thought—expressed as an interpretation—that was different from what he anticipated, particularly when I suggested a link between an emotional state and its somatic expression. These encounters, when Sam was unable to follow what I was telling him or, better yet, be two steps ahead of me, would leave him feeling small, empty and alone—and in contact with his own terror, murderous rage and self-hatred. The self-hatred related to his not being an "A student" in the analysis; the rage was directed at me for having exposed it; and the terror was connected to his fear of "going crazy" if life, including the analysis, didn't play out like a computer game that he could be assured of controlling. In his identification with the *Blade Runner* replicants, this would mean that something in his programming had snapped, leaving him feeling vulnerable and exposed. Sam eloquently expressed this dilemma in the middle of his seventh year of treatment. He had become quite emotional the previous day after I addressed his propensity to hide behind an omnipotent shell to avoid the risk of being exposed as different than others:

PATIENT: Part of me is afraid to be who I am or acknowledge who I am because it's crappy and bleak … I feel unlikeable, unlovable, and untouchable in the Indian caste system way … This needs to be dealt with—ignored, changed, whatever. When I was feeling crappy yesterday and started to think about it, I got wrenched out of the feeling. This is uncomfortable so do I want to go through it again? Yesterday was painful; it wasn't fun.

ANALYST: I think you want me to know how scary it is for you to be in contact with these painful feelings.

PATIENT: Sometimes, when I'm sick and can't come in, I feel relieved. That speaks to what you're saying. But, hiding is hard work; it's fatiguing. So much here is painful—yesterday, today, other days. It's painful. It sucks. Of all people, you should be prepared for who I am and to be able to handle me … I wonder if I learned at an early age to chop off pieces of this and stuff it inside.My hypothesis is that when Sam feels uncontained, he becomes terrified of fragmenting or falling to bits, much like what occurred after his sister Carrie's suicide. This fear is coupled with his lack of confidence in being able to learn from experience. According to Bion (1962), when the infant has had sufficient opportunity to communicate his experience through projective identification and to internalize his mother's capacity to tolerate and think about him—i.e., when he feels contained—he is able to experience a more sturdy sense of himself and his objects, facilitating a degree of tolerance of, and openness to, experience, both internally and externally. This forms the basis of a capacity to learn from the emotional impact of life, what Bion refers to as "learning from experience". Without the experience of containment, Sam never learned to deal with those feelings or any of the other dangers of being fully human; and, like the *Blade Runner* replicants, he both hoped to pass as human and feared the consequences if he did.

Shortly after the session referenced above, Sam experienced an episode of severe hypoglycemia that resulted in a visit to the ER, and in his leaving a physician he had seen for years and whom he experienced as uncaring. Sam found a new physician at another clinic, and in working with him he lost more than 75 pounds over an 18-month period. I sensed a complex internal shift coincident with the change in his appearance. He had a greater sense of agency as a result of having stayed with the diet and having accomplished his goal. In the transference–countertransference relationship the "old physician" represents me when I'm unable to contain my patient's primitive anxieties, while he is able to experience me as the "new physician" when I am able to contain and transform his terror about being alive so that we might function as an analytic couple.

Unfortunately, there was an unanticipated downside to Sam's weight loss. He began having intrusive thoughts of stabbing or maiming his wife and, in our sessions, he told me that he was having thoughts of hurting and/or stalking me. This calamitous turn of events led me to speculate that what I thought of as Sam's "wall of fat" had, in phantasy, functioned as a kind of somatic bunker that had protected him from falling to bits in much the same way that the psychic bunker, his reliance on the virtual reality, had done. Now his psychotic core was exposed, and again he was caught in an intolerable conflict between wanting to be seen for who he is and fearing the consequences of visibility. This time Sam was started on antipsychotic medication, which proved effective in diminishing his intrusive thoughts but carried with it the side effect of increased appetite and weight gain. As Sam became terrified by the return of the psychotic symptoms he had struggled against since adolescence he abandoned the diet, regaining most of the weight he had lost in less than six months.

In the analysis, I have sensed that Sam struggles between identifying himself as a character he creates and "runs" (as a human bioengineer "runs" a replicant) and exposing himself to the (unpredictable) myriad of emotions associated with being human. In the sessions which feel most alive to me, Sam is spontaneous; he associates freely, and feels less need to anticipate how I will respond to him. In sessions driven by destructive narcissistic impulses, he tends to repeat material, often embellished with bits of what I have previously said to him in response—thus forestalling any new and unanticipated dangers. Sadly for both of us, as soon as a new thought or a creative action evokes a sense of aliveness in him, the part of him committed to maintaining psychic equilibrium shuts it down for fear of his falling apart.

A sign of hope: the capacity to dream

In a long analysis such as this, the analyst faces the challenge of having to stay as close as possible to the patient's material while still maintaining a perspective of the journey thus far traversed. I believe that one can best accomplish this dual perspective through a careful tracking of the patient's dreams. Sam brought in one significant dream at the beginning of the analysis, but then no dreams at all for several years. My speculation on this has led me to believe that exposing himself to me through his dreams was particularly frightening because doing so would rob him of being able to stay one step ahead in the transference–countertransference. However, over the long years of his treatment, Sam has gradually become able to experience me as a trustworthy object who can, at least at times, provide empathic containment. This has gradually allowed him to crawl out of his psychic bunker and to let him be in touch with himself and with humanity. Furthermore, as Sam has become less terrified, his competition with me has subsided, and for this reason too he has been able, little by little, to invite me into the theater of his internal world. Thus, I will end this section with two dreams: one from the eighth year of treatment and the second that is more recent. Sam's nascent psychic development is apparent in the contrast between the two dreams.

Dream #1. Sam brought in the following dream fragments after a session in which he related something he felt shameful about, and subsequently felt criticized by me:

> In the first dream fragment, Sam described being by himself in a desolate, barren landscape with no orienting objects—no mountains, no trees, not even a horizon line separating the ground from the sky. He said that he woke up and went back to sleep, whereupon he had the same dream.

> After waking and going back to sleep a third time he had a different dream. In this one, he was by himself in his house and was opening a letter that had come for him. However, once he opened the envelope, he found a blank piece of paper and felt frustrated and anxious. I queried him for more details and the only one that occurred to him was that the letter in the dream was from me.

The first fragment describes where Sam was in his analysis at the time—alone, in new terrain and without anything to orient to—while the second fragment seemed to locate him in the transference: wanting desperately for me to send him concrete instructions and, instead, feeling disappointed and enraged when I didn't fulfill this phantasy of a continuous feed from my brain to his. It is also possible to think about this dream as representing Sam's growth toward containment: He can send me his projections, but has not yet learned how to make use of my processing and transformation of them. Ultimately, he will become able to see me as a good object able to receive his projections (*beta elements*) and transform them into dream thoughts (*alpha elements*) through the process of reverie.

Here is the second dream:

> My dream was about Carrie. I was older than her. We were in a foreign country, like Pakistan, and our father was with us. We were near a hill or sand dune and Carrie was playing in it at the base. I'm standing near her. The sand starts to shift, like an avalanche, and she's digging in it with a toy shovel. I don't know if she caused it or whether her digging is helping to slow it down. She becomes buried, all but her lower legs. The sand is still coming down but, instead of pulling her out, I ran. I made it out but other people got trapped. Some people got pulled out and others crawled out but Carrie doesn't make it. She dies. There was a ceremony, or memorial, for people who died or got hurt. I walked by and they gave me a dirty look because I didn't say "Sorry." I got pissed off and started crying. Then I woke up.

As we began exploring this dream together, Sam told me that the earthquake was actually more like a tsunami that "wipes things out as if they never existed." This allowed us to consider together that his inability to mourn his sister had left him feeling as if she had never existed—that, like the shifting sand in the dream, he had buried the fact of her death as well as his feelings surrounding it. The last element in the dream, Sam's survivor guilt, was new territory for us. Sam drew a parallel between the way Carrie in the dream caused the sand to shift while trying to dig out of it with a toy shovel, and her having shot herself in response to command hallucinations.

Theoretical considerations

Three related theoretical concepts were helpful to me in my clinical work with Sam: Bion's notion of containment; the inaccessibility of mourning when containment has failed; and the resulting defensive recourse to psychotic encapsulation. Finally, I will note a technical observation by Betty Joseph that I have found pertinent in this analysis.

Containment

I have noted above Bion's hypothesis about how the mother's metabolizing of her infant's distress signals makes unbearable pain bearable. When maternal reverie *is* available, the experience of containment forms an intuitive background within which the infant's distress signals are understood and addressed, transforming what is "sensed" into "thought". When the mother cannot acknowledge and contain her baby's distress, however, the baby is left with what Bion called *nameless dread* (1962, p. 96)—an unnamed, unacknowledged, unbounded, and hence fearsome quantum of anxiety. I believe that my patient's primary maternal object was not able to help him contain his early anxieties sufficiently, and that in order to psychically survive overwhelming trauma, he developed psychotic defenses.

In calling Sam's fluctuating states of mind *psychotic*, I am using Bion's (1957, p. 44) definition of the term. Bion hypothesized that all humans have a psychotic core, which remains quiescent unless the individual experiences overwhelming stress or trauma. He ascribed to it four essential features: (1) a preponderance of destructive impulses so great that even the impulse to love is suffused by them and turned to sadism; (2) a hatred of reality, internal and external, which is extended to all that makes for awareness of it; (3) a dread of imminent annihilation; and (4) a premature and precipitate formation of object relations, foremost among which is the transference, whose thinness is in marked contrast with the tenacity with which they are maintained. According to Robert Oelsner (personal communication, 2017), Bion was fond of playing with contradiction in his writings. With this in mind, we may assume that he used "thinness" to mean the same as fragile, easily breakable and highly unstable, which is in contrast with tenacity. Hence, the psychotic transference in its fragility (thinness) firmly (tenaciously) grips the analyst and won't let loose. All of these features were prominent in my patient.

Theoretically, there are two contributing factors to any individual's lack of frustration tolerance: innate disposition, and the failure of the containing environment. I do not know Sam's mother; but, as I stated earlier, my clinical experience with him suggests that she was significantly absent as a containing object in his early years. However, it is also possible to conjecture (as Sam did himself in his comment above about being "too nurtured") that Sam started life believing that he was special, and thus exempt from waiting and having to tolerate discomfort and frustration. Here, I'm referring to *internal phantasy*, as defined by Isaacs (1948) as unconscious mental processes which function as defenses against anxiety. These are believed to start at birth, if not before. In either case or both, Sam would have borne a heavy burden of frustration, which he had to process without recourse to the normal containing processes of projection and introjection. Thus impeded, I contend, my patient was unable to develop an ego capable of psychic development, leaving him vulnerable to relying on the psychotic defenses that Bion describes.

Bion's way of differentiating between the psychotic and non-psychotic parts of the personality is also pertinent. With sufficient containment, a binding takes place between the psychotic and non-psychotic parts, ensuring that regression to psychosis occurs only under extreme stress. Without containment, however, the psychotic part of the personality is "cut up, split into minute fragments and then, using projective identification, expelled from the personality, rendering the patient unable to tolerate reality, both internal and external" (Bion, 1957/1967, p. 38). But this remedy creates another problem. Having rid himself of the psychic pain associated with conscious awareness of internal and external reality, the patient achieves a state within which he feels neither alive nor dead: a psychic stalemate. I believe that a widening of the gap between the psychotic and the non-psychotic parts of my patient's personality began during infancy, were exposed for the first time after Carrie's suicide, and then again after his weight loss.

Mourning

Along with the other psychic deficits it creates, lack of containment during infancy renders the infant, and later the adult, unable to mourn. Freud described the process of mourning in great detail, emphasizing that the work of mourning is the painful facing of the *reality* of loss. He distinguishes this from melancholia, in which what is lost is not experienced as the loved object, but as the self, or a part of the self.

> The melancholic displays something else besides what is lacking in mourning—an extraordinary diminution of his self-regard, an impoverishment of his ego on a grand scale. In mourning it is the world which has become poor and empty; in melancholia it is the ego itself. (Freud, 1917, p. 245)

When successful, the process of mourning leads to an acknowledgment of the loss and consequent enrichment of the mourner. John Steiner (1990) elaborates on Freud's concept of melancholia in his discussion of why mourning is difficult for individuals who are entrapped in pathological organizations. He says that the capacity to acknowledge the reality of the loss is what leads to the differentiation of self from object, and is therefore the critical issue that determines whether normal or pathological mourning will ensue. Completion of the mourning process requires relinquishing the fantasy of control over the object, and the denial of reality that this fantasy entails. Successful mourning means that the bereft individual has to face his inability to protect, and to possess, the object in phantasy. This is a painful process and one fraught with conflict, which makes it difficult to pursue to its conclusion without a sturdy internal object in place.

When the normal process of mourning is impeded, the patient will attempt to deny the loss by trying to possess and preserve the object, primarily through identification with it. This identification with the object implies to the mourner that if the object dies, he must die with it. Conversely, if he survives then the reality of the loss must be denied. This is precisely the fine line between aliveness and deadness that Sam has attempted to navigate most of his adult life.

While Steiner proposes that a psychic retreat may be a *consequence* of pathological mourning, Franco De Masi believes that such withdrawal, which begins in infancy, is instead the *condition* that prepares the ground for the later psychotic explosion, which finds its fuel in the retreat itself; that is, in emotional detachment and dissociation from both external and psychic reality. He says:

> My thought is that psychotic withdrawal is primitive and is established precociously in infancy, when the child "loses" his mother. Indeed, withdrawal, in which the patient lives for long periods and which progressively deteriorates his contact with emotional and relational reality, cancels the experience and memory of the trauma. (De Masi, 2006, p. 795)

Autistic encapsulation

Sydney Klein's ideas about autistic defenses also helped me understand how the lack of early containment contributed to my patient's psychic retreat in response to the traumatic losses he experienced. Klein described autistic phenomena as being characterized by "an almost impenetrable encapsulation of part of the personality, mute and implacable resistance to change, and a lack of real emotional contact either with themselves or with the analyst" (1980, p. 400). He added the following:

> The autistic defense is primarily due to the avoidance of the pain caused by the intensity of the fear of death and disintegration caused by the absence of the containing nipple or breast. This surfaces … not only at weekend and holiday separations but every time the patient makes a step forward and becomes more separate … [Patients like this] use various projective processes to deflect painful emotions either into other people, including the analyst, or into their own bodies. (1980, pp. 400–401)

Technical considerations

I have found Betty Joseph's (1976) work enormously valuable in understanding the glacial pace of this analysis, and some of its technical challenges. She describes patients whose struggle to maintain their psychic equilibrium comes at the cost of denying the psychic realities of time and loss. She notes that this phenomenon is most apparent in the patient's experience of breaks in the treatment.

> In such patients ... holidays and gaps can be non-experienced up to a point, because such patients retreat into their world and keep up a type of internal euphoric relationship with the analyst, which is quite different from an internal relationship based on the introjection of an object who has been experienced as physically real and valued, loved or hated. (1976, p. 95)

I experienced this phenomenon repeatedly in my work with Sam. Although less pervasive than it was previously, for a long time he would feign surprise when I reminded him of an upcoming break, seeming to "forget" that he had been informed about it previously. He would typically miss the Monday session after a break, returning on Tuesday with my interpretation about the missed session already formulated in his mind, as a way of denying any sense of loss or separation between us.

Conclusion

One profound aspect of being alive is the capacity to feel empathy for oneself and for others, as well as the capacity to accept the limits—including mortality—of our humanity. We learn these capacities through the experience of being empathized with and accepted, especially in the context of containment and maternal reverie. In the quote I offered as my epigraph, the replicant leader Roy Batty empathically shares a moment of aesthetic communion with blade runner Rick Deckard after sparing Deckard's life at the cost of his own. For me, this quote captures the exquisite paradox of feeling alive: It requires the capacity to imagine and to mourn one's death. The fact that this moment is shared between beings who had previously been mortal enemies contributes to its profundity.

All of the authors whom I have cited and Sam's clinical material suggest that the capacity for empathy—for oneself and for others—is impeded when strong feeling cannot be contained, and when reliance on omnipotent, narcissistic or psychotic defense mechanisms prevails instead. As was the case with Sam, patients who rely on a form of autistic encapsulation, or the creation of a psychic bunker, maintain psychic equilibrium at the cost of losing not only a sense of aliveness but also the feeling of existing as part of humanity. The replicants in *Blade Runner* fight to extend their lives, and feel angry, demoralized and bereft (particularly in the case of Batty) when they are unable to do so. In contrast, Sam retreated from his life in late adolescence when he found himself unable to mourn the loss of his sister. In the film, we see the four-year life span of the replicants giving their lives a sense of poignancy, even urgency, while for most of his adult life, Sam devoted himself to the nihilistic notion that "life is meaningless" as a way to maintain his psychic equilibrium. However, as Sam is slowly developing the capacity to mourn his many losses, he has also begun the process of reclaiming his life.

References

Bion, W.R. (1957). Differentiation of the psychotic from the non-psychotic personalities. *Second Thoughts: Selected Papers on Psycho-Analysis*. London: Heinemann, 1967, 43–64. Reprint: Northvale, NJ: Aronson, 1983.

Bion, W.R. (1959). Attacks on linking. *Second Thoughts: Selected Papers on Psychoanalysis*. London: Heinemann, 1967, 93–109. Reprint: Northvale, NJ: Aronson, 1983.

Bion, W.R. (1962). *Learning from Experience*. London: Karnac.

Bion, W.R. (1962a). A theory of thinking. *Second Thoughts: Selected Papers on Psychonalysis*. London: Heinemann, 1967, 110–119. Reprint: Northvale, NJ: Aronson, 1983.

Blade Runner: The Final Cut. (2007). [DVD]. Los Angeles: Warner Bros. Inc., 117 minutes. Excerpt offered courtesy of Warner Bros. Entertainment Inc. Screenplay by Hampton Fancher and David Peoples, reprinted with permission.

De Masi, F. (2006). Psychotic withdrawal and the overthrow of psychic reality. *International Journal of Psychoanalysis*, 87: 789–807.

Freud, S. (1917). Mourning and melancholia. *Standard Edition 14*: 237–258.

Isaacs, S. (1948). On the nature and function of phantasy. *International Journal of Psychoanalysis*, 29: 73–97; republished in M. Klein, P. Heimann, S. Isaacs & J. Riviere (eds.), *Developments in Psychoanalysis*. London: Hogarth Press, 1952.

Joseph, B. (1976). Towards the experiencing of psychic pain. *Do I Dare Disturb the Universe? A Memorial to Wilfred R. Bion*, J.S. Grotstein (ed.). Beverly Hills, CA: Caesura Press, 1981.

Klein, S. (1980). Autistic phenomena in neurotic patients. *International Journal of Psychoanalysis*, 61: 395–402.

Steiner, J. (1990). Pathological organizations as obstacles to mourning: The role of unbearable guilt. *International Journal of Psychoanalysis*, 71: 87–94.

Szykierski, D. (2010). The traumatic roots of containment: The evolution of Bion's metapsychology. *Psychoanalytic Quarterly*, 79(4): 935–968.

Winnicott, D.W. (1965). *The Maturational Processes and the Facilitating Environment: Studies in the Theory of Emotional Development*. London: Hogarth Press.

Chapter 8

Trauma and embodied memory

Marilyn Rifkin

"I'm panicking," says Ms. D. It is near the end of the session. She has just started to use the couch after 16 years of "sitting up" in a psychoanalytic therapy that consisted of contact often no more than once, and occasionally twice, per week. For a long time, Ms. D had been almost inaccessible—a patient who experienced her feelings on a concrete (desymbolized) level and had been very hard to reach. She is now talking of coming to treatment more often—she would eventually like a full analysis of three times per week. This, to me, seems nothing short of a miracle, given what we had started with so many years before.

"Can you say anything more about the panic?" I ask.

"I don't know," she responds. There is a terror in her voice. "I'm beginning to feel raw and exposed," she says, finally. She sits up.

"Raw and exposed." These are important words. They are words that have developed significant meaning between Ms. D and me in terms of memories that have just recently emerged—memories of being overstimulated at a pediatrician's office where she underwent repeated invasive vaginal examinations due to what was diagnosed as a congenital problem that had caused enuresis in childhood. But perhaps even more significantly, other memories have surfaced that have produced a fuller picture of a depressed, narcissistically fragile mother who was emotionally labile though psychically "dead" and who, at best, treated Ms. D as a narcissistic extension of herself—a self-object to be "owned", "controlled" and "managed" but not accepted as separate and whole.

What led to Ms. D's recall of aspects of past trauma—and her willingness to lie on the couch—is the topic of this chapter. Specifically, I will show that in order to understand the dissociative states of Ms. D, it was essential to decode the language of her body and to connect it with visualizations, images and verbalizations in the transference (and countertransference). Such decoding has its roots in the concept of "embodied memory", a concept described by Leuzinger-Bohleber (2008) and others, which offers an understanding of the way early trauma is remembered through bodily experience. In my work with Ms. D, by observing, in detail, the bodily sensations and bodily communication in the analytic relationship (both in Ms. D and in myself) we were able to decode the intensity of affects and fantasies which seemingly matched original traumatic interaction that had been split off, encapsulated, if you will, and therefore unintegrated within her psychic life. This "decoding", at first, presented as discrete aspects of traumatic experience which were slowly transformed into symbolic language, ultimately offering an understanding and integration of the trauma into Ms. D's own personal history and identity. Through this painstaking process, the trauma came more to life within the transference/countertransference matrix. Ultimately, the reconstruction of original traumatic experience proved indispensable in helping Ms. D to understand the "language of the body" as it related to the heretofore gaps in the comprehension of her internal experience. The emotional wounds and vulnerability expressed through her body were viewed as the "signs of her specific traumatic history" (Leuzinger-Bohleber, 2008). Ultimately they were emotionally accepted, understood and mentalized—transmuted into a symbolized form in which they could be worked with on a more verbal, metaphoric level.

Ms. D

Ms. D is a 48-year-old married woman and mother of a 12-year-old daughter. When she began treatment she was 32 and single, but was married two years later. She is well-educated and has a career in the field of child development.

Ms. D presented from the outset as bright and well-spoken, despite a significant depressive affect that seemed indelibly "written" on her face. With pale skin and deep circles under her eyes, she always (until recently) looked as though she had been crying copious amounts of tears on a daily basis. However, one of her presenting complaints was that she couldn't cry—and that she, indeed, was alexythemic. She couldn't readily access and/or distinguish her feelings. What she was most aware of was a sense of panic and desperation.

Ms. D was born the youngest of three children. Her sister and brother are 8 and 6 years her senior, respectively. Her father, with whom she says she felt a "kind of" closeness, worked a lot and was physically absent during most of her childhood. He died 25 years ago of a heart ailment. Ms. D's mother is still alive, but she and mother are almost entirely estranged.

As noted, mother has been depicted as depressed and narcissistically driven. It seems that mother was emotionally labile and, at the same time, lived in a world of her own and so there was little or no true emotional access for Ms. D. As infant research has shown, an infant is severely affected when, for example, mother either avoids or aggressively pursues eye contact, or when she neutralizes her own facial expression as an experimental condition (Bach, 2002a). Ms. D and I now speculate that her mother was one who would have aggressively pursued eye contact, and so Ms. D withdrew in order to avoid mother's intrusiveness.

From what Ms. D can now remember, her mother always wanted Ms. D to be "a perfect child." Mother's expectations of Ms. D were high. Of particular significance in relation to Ms. D's secondary enuresis is the fact that mother reportedly had tried to toilet train Ms. D before she had reached the age of one year. One can only imagine how Ms. D's mother had reacted when Ms. D began wetting her bed at the age of eight.

I conjecture that mother's intrusiveness and narcissism did not allow Ms. D adequate "room" to develop a mind of her own (Bach, 2002b). Ms. D could not make sufficient sense of mother's mind as a separate entity, and so she never came to understand her own mind. Confused and disoriented, Ms. D admits that she has had difficulty making sense of the world of emotions and of relatedness with others throughout her life. She has never felt completely at home in the world, and has felt alone and unmoored.

I previously wrote about Ms. D where I used a clinical vignette to illustrate how the pressures for enactment were intensified by her "hatred of reality" (Rifkin, 2013). Given her history, it is no surprise (in retrospect) that Ms. D, as a patient, preferred a "pre-thinking state" of mind characterized by concreteness and feelings of omnipotence. From the outset, she was not always able to separate "real" experiences from the "not real". As noted, her feelings were mostly non-distinguishable. When feelings were discerned at all, they were described as bodily sensations. Sadness felt like "burning in the eyes." Anger felt like "warmth" in the face.

As treatment unfolded, there was, as Jodi Davies (2004) has put it, a "malignancy" infusing the transference–countertransference relationship, a malignancy that did not allow for the creation of "analytic space." A quasi-erotized, sadomasochistic transference became a central theme. I became the object of Ms. D's painful desire—her craving—even while she dated, and eventually married, her husband. She often told me she thought about me all the time and "couldn't wait" to see me, and that she "couldn't get enough" of me. On the other hand, she felt tortured by the power of her longing and, in sessions, would often shut down and seemed unreachable. Her desperate longing reflected strong dependency needs and disturbances in self–other differentiation (as well as an identification, perhaps, with her needy, narcissistically driven mother). While I had cursory ideas about Ms. D's troubles, she remained a patient whom I mostly felt overwhelmed and confused by.

What I was aware of was her powerful ambivalence, which manifested in an oscillation between an intense desire for closeness and an equally intense need for distance. It soon became apparent that Ms. D either held me in the utmost esteem (while denigrating herself) or vice versa. These oscillating self states were disturbing for me and for her. They were difficult to manage, and obviously prevented a more symbolic way of working. Ms. D felt torture; I felt tortured.

Sadomasochistic pathology, according to Sheldon Bach (2002a), often follows a variety of childhood traumata which leads to an intensification of annihilation and/or castration anxiety. In Bach's understanding of sadomasochism, relationships with primary objects are oriented predominantly toward pain rather than toward pleasure, and that what feels longed for, reassuring and familiar is some variety of painful rather than pleasurable interaction. This idea truly captures the nature of Ms. D's interactions with me perfectly.

There were many topics that Ms. D delineated as "off-limits" in our sessions and if I "slipped" and made mention of any of these, there was hell to pay, often in the form of attacks on linking (Bion, 1959). These destructive attacks prevented any link between emotion and reason. For example, Ms. D could not tolerate my making any mention of her father and/or his death. She accepted the notion that she had never adequately mourned, but she vehemently worked at shutting out reality, preempting any attempt at identifying and working through her feelings. Whenever I alluded to his death in any way Ms. D would sometimes shut down completely and become mute, closing her eyes, breathing heavily and, seemingly, writhing in pain. At other times, she would glare at me with murderous eyes and would take a snipe at me verbally. On these occasions, she would accuse me of criticizing her and/or trying to hurt her. "I told you I will not talk about this," she would say in a menacing tone. Later on in the treatment, she forbade me from speaking about her mother, and any slip up on my part was met with some variety of the same reactions.

Often enough, Ms. D and I experienced these episodes as agonizing. These were instances of absolute despair, sessions where we both felt that we couldn't go on any longer. When Ms. D would threaten, at times, to terminate, I would feel a welcome sense of relief. On several occasions, however, Ms. D would talk about a fantasy of jumping out the window in front of me (my office is on the 25th floor). With a spark of glee in her eye, she would note that she would happily turn back as she was going out the window, in order to enjoy the look of "horror" on my face as she fell to her death—the ultimate in manic triumph! Ah, I would think to myself, would she see "horror" or delight on my face? Though conscious, at times, of my own hatred, I mostly tried to ignore and avoid it (Rifkin, 2013).

We seemed in a sadomasochistic stalemate. She was either passively silent and/or "obedient" or sadistic, and I would experience myself as either a sadistic abuser or a victim. If I remained silent, Ms. D would feel that I was depriving her. If I spoke, it was experienced as an attack and/or a condemnation. The boundaries between us would often become confused—and confusing. Sometimes it was difficult to ascertain who said what to whom. Indeed, I would often feel as if I was going out of my mind—and I often worried that Ms. D would have a psychotic break.

I felt at a loss as to how to proceed. At the urging of a colleague, I began using a technique that Sheldon Bach has recommended: I allowed Ms. D to hear the reasoning behind my thinking, and also allowed her "to witness my mind at work in the process of free-associating or making formulations" (Bach, 2011, p. 52). This was a way of helping to create boundaries while establishing meaningful links. I would speak to Ms. D about aspects of my feeling and thinking process in relation to what I understood was happening in a given session. In other words, I talked to her about how my mind worked in relation to my experience of her and how I reached conclusions about her.

I was not always able to utilize this technique with Ms. D because I so often became entangled in a massive knot of projective and introjective identification. But whenever I was able to pull myself out of the maelstrom, I would talk about my process, and Ms. D would become calm and thoughtful. It seemed that such remarks opened up just enough psychic space to allow for a move toward self-reflection and mentalization (Fonagy & Target, 1998).

Given her strengthening selfhood, the stakes in many ways became higher. Ms. D grew more in touch with her destructive impulses, and in turn would readily revert to a more primitive, "pre-thinking" state of mind.

Despite some progress, Ms. D continued to hate the reality of separateness and the accompanying feelings of helplessness, envy and rage. My ability to think continued to be a threat and she, in turn, would continue to attack my ability to think and process. In order to fend off this sensory bombardment, I would collude by escaping into a similar pre-thinking state. Through this ongoing enactment, an impasse was created. I eventually found my way out of the impasse one day by admitting to Ms. D that, at times, I hated her. She hadn't been paying me for a while and, when I asked about it, she became defensive in her "split off" way. Her face was a blank and she told me repeatedly that she couldn't pay until she received money from her insurance company. Meanwhile, she knew very well that my policy was not to take insurance assignment. In the past, she had paid punctually. I tried to help her "see" that something else—something emotionally meaningful—was responsible for her not paying, but she "attacked" the connection by impassively repeating that she had to wait for the insurance money and why didn't I know that. She talked seemingly "in circles" and all the while her face was blank, impassive. The more logic I used, the more she seemingly "attacked" *my* ability to think, and I became confused—and angry. She remained calm and I was bubbling inside with venom. She read the look of rage on my face. "You hate me," she said, finally. And I answered that, yes, at that moment I did hate her, but that I didn't always. She immediately relaxed and we were able to come up with a payment plan that worked for her. She came alive and our minds began to work together.

This was another example of Bach's recommendation for the analyst to describe her own internal process to the patient. This form of limited self-disclosure truly seemed a turning point within the session and beyond. We had been able to find our way out of the impasse. My admission, and her response to it, deepened our analytic work from then on. It created some space for us to think together about hateful feelings and fantasies. The labeling of my own hatred gave Ms. D some room (and permission) to explore her own (as yet) un-metabolized hatred. A "container" had formed which facilitated a greater sense of safety as Ms. D continued to struggle with raw affect within the dyad.

But by no means did Ms. D feel safe enough. There was still a plethora of moments where words could not be accessed and Ms. D would revert to a more concrete, embodied, action-oriented way of coping in her sessions.

And so, despite the "breakthrough", Ms. D continued to be a patient who frequently struggled with "concrete" unmetabolized states of consciousness. We both continued to feel stuck in our understanding of her inner world as it manifested within the transference/countertransference matrix. Enactments continued to abound. It seemed evident to both of us that there was significant underlying trauma in her past, but Ms. D continued to elucidate few clear memories, as is so typical in patients with traumatic histories. Because she remembered so little of her childhood, there seemed to be few stable representations to utilize and she had virtually no access to her dreams.

The embodied dimension

Ellman and Goodman have stressed that overwhelming affect is often the result of early trauma and inevitably leads to enactments that tend to bypass symbolic narrative. These enactments are repeatedly communicated through various modes of action that remain fixed. Labeling affect in the enacted dimension "brings clarity and further differentiation to traumatic experience and to the associated unconscious fantasies" (Ellman & Goodman, 2012, p. 59). As I've already shown, Ms. D often communicated through modes of action and I would often get pulled into the act. Such enactments clearly had enormous implications in terms of identifying and understanding the underlying trauma.

In their work on trauma, Marianne Leuzinger-Bohleber and Werner Bohleber have shown that the concept of "embodied memory" is often helpful in understanding that early trauma is remembered by the body in a more specific way than in merely understanding procedural memories (meaning mechanical or bodily skills) in the transference (Leuzinger-Bohleber, 2008; Bohleber, 2010).

The enacted dimension for Ms. D often involved an embodied dimension. There was a significant split between what Ms. D verbalized and what she expressed through her body. For instance, she would look at me with an angry face but be completely unaware of it when I pointed it out to her. As previously noted, at times her facial expression would seem incredibly sinister—menacing, reflective of a murderous rage, and I could feel the hairs on my arms standing on end. At other times, she would sit with her legs pressed together tightly and with her hands covering her vaginal area. She was unaware of this also. This last aspect, in particular, seemed obviously linked to the heightened state of sexual arousal she admittedly often experienced in my presence. I became aware that I was unconsciously shutting myself down in reaction to these nonverbal, embodied messages. In order to find my way "in", I found it helpful to talk to Ms. D about her body language and facial expressions.

As a result of my comments on her body's communications, Ms. D began to remember more about her past. We began to focus on the various split-off aspects of her internal world and there slowly emerged layers of trauma in her past, including the memories of the frequent visits to the pediatrician from ages 7 to 12 for the ongoing urological problems. Ms. D soon remembered intrusive vaginal examinations that were both exciting and painful, as well as one minor procedure to help correct a genetic anomaly. Previously unformulated experience slowly began to be metabolized and understood. What unfolded was a typical pattern: She would have a "good" session (where she opened up and let things "flow"), followed by a "bad" one during which she was flooded with anxiety, became dissociated and, therefore, "out of reach". In these "bad" sessions, she continued to have trouble naming her feelings, although, in general, she was becoming more and more reflective. It became apparent to me that Ms. D's "shutting down" in the sessions was a reaction to the "flow" of the previous session and was linked to her need to "hold in" terrifying affect, in the same way that she had to "hold in" her urge to urinate.

Another enactment

A compelling enactment in one critical session (described below) involved a glaring transgression on my part, and brought to life aspects of trauma that related, on one level, to the dramatic emotional abandonment that Ms. D felt with her mother throughout her childhood—and even on into adulthood. In the enactment, I lost control and broke the frame by responding to a phone text during the session—metaphorically "peeing" where and when I wasn't supposed to, and I immediately felt humiliated and exposed. In response, Ms. D withdrew and shut down. She went "dead" and stopped speaking (much the way her mother might have acted when Ms. D had an "accident" and wet her bed). Despite the "deadness", she nevertheless seemed in touch with a powerful anxiety that must have felt threatening to her very being—a state of unspeakable horror, a nameless dread. This was written on her face and in her body language, and my only recourse was to comment on how her body was speaking to me. What evolved within that session was a visible shift where the "split" was resolved (at least momentarily) and Ms. D came back to life and to me.

Ms. D had come into her session on the day of the enactment in a somewhat anxious state, although she was extremely eager to tell me that she had had recent contact with her mother with whom she had not been speaking for months. "My mother sounded different to me," she said. "Her voice was high-pitched. She sounded weak." We explored what that "weakness" meant to Ms. D. She began to describe the fear of her mother dying. "I don't know how I'll deal with it. Part of me will feel relieved. Part of me will feel upset and worried about the intensity of my upset." We talked about her fear of her sadness, her fear of losing control and crying—and feeling alone with it. This led to the feelings she had when her father died—how she couldn't process it, how she had to shut down. (In all of this, I must admit, I was having a hard time with my own feelings of sadness. My husband had died some months before, and I was still grieving.) All of a sudden I heard the familiar buzz of my iPhone, indicating a text message. I had "forgotten" to shut the phone off. I glanced and saw that the text was from a patient who had just given birth, that day, to her second child. I texted back "congratulations" on the spot.

Ms. D asked in an affectless voice what the interruption to our session was all about and I told her, briefly. She withdrew immediately and I, in turn, felt a sense of shame and guilt. It was a bodily sensation. I felt, for a moment, naked and exposed. Meanwhile, there was a look of malevolence on Ms. D's face but she was dissociated. I spoke to her but I could not reach her. Facial expressions of menacing rage alternated with a horrifying (for me) blankness. Meanwhile, I remained flabbergasted at my own dissociated behavior. I realized that I had moved to "life" instead of "death" in the scenario for some obvious and personal reasons of my own, as well as from what was being unconsciously "projected" by Ms. D and repeated within the session.

"You are angry and you have every right to be angry. That was wrong of me to do," I said. Ms. D remained silent for several minutes more, before she spoke.

"I don't know what I'm feeling right now," she finally replied. Her voice was flat—she seemed very far away.

"Let's try to talk about it," I said.

"What is there to talk about? What's done is done," she said. She then went silent again, all the while looking at me blankly. Soon I saw glimmers of a hatred fused with incredible sadness on her face. I did not want to let the moment pass without saying something.

"Your face is now speaking to me. You are furious. You are sad."

"Maybe," she said. "I just don't know. It's confusing." And then: "That was wrong of you to do."

Then, more silence—a deadly silence.

"You've just gone dead on me again," I said.

She shrugged.

More silence—more deadness. "You've gone dead on me. Now you are the one who is dead, not your mother or your father."

"And you are dead," she said. A chill ran up my spine. We sat in silence, again, for several minutes more.

Finally, I confessed to her what I thought was going on in me in the enactment: "You know I think that when you were talking about the possible death of your mother—and also your father's death—I felt sad about my husband. I think I answered that text to avoid that sadness."

Ms. D came back to life just then. "Thank you for saying that," she said. And at that moment, she squeezed her legs together.

"You are squeezing your legs together."

"I am not aware of that."

"Memories of being at the doctor's office?"

More silence and then:

"Yes. Alone in the doctor's office."

"Alone?"

"Yes. I felt alone. My mother was there but I felt she wasn't there."

"It was like she was dead?"

"Yes."

"She abandoned you?"

"Yes."

"Like I abandoned you just now?"

"Yes. When I needed you most." Tears welled up in her eyes. "That makes a lot of sense to me," she said. "At that moment, before you picked up the phone, I was feeling really sad—and panicky—and I felt you didn't care. I felt abandoned."

"So perhaps you wanted to kill me."

"Perhaps."

As many authors have noted, countertransference often can be utilized to identify aspects of an enactment that can then help the patient enter into a more symbolizing mode (Ellman & Goodman, 2012). Subsequent to this enactment, Ms. D and I were able to build on our understanding of herself and her early history. We began to understand her early childhood where her mother was absent emotionally and where her father (who was much more alive and vital to her) was physically absent due to a grueling work schedule. Ms. D recalled many instances of fearing that she would lose both parents, reflective of her unconscious rage-filled murderous fantasies against them. We also talked more about her enuresis, her own and her mother's probable reaction to it, and the trauma of the medical treatment. We talked about rage and exposure, excitement and shame. We talked about how Ms. D needed to "go dead", as it were, in order to bear the pain, humiliation—as well as the sexual excitement she felt when the doctor examined her. Ms. D revealed that, while the doctor hadn't really done "anything morally wrong," she, nevertheless, had felt that she had been "sexually molested" by him. Obviously, there was so much more to understand about all of this.

A few weeks after the enactment, Ms. D came in and said, "I've been thinking a lot about this couch." "What about it?" I asked. "I think I'm ready to try it out. I want to go deeper. I want to understand more. I think I'm ready to do that."

Discussion

According to "embodied memory" theory, memory is a constructive and adaptive process through which the whole organism interacts with the environment and connects past experience with corresponding new situations through sensorimotor coordination "in a continual process of recategorization" (Leuzinger-Bohleber & Pfeifer, 2002). Neuroscientific data concerning the construction of memories leads some to conclude that memories are narrative constructions containing gaps that arise as a result of forgetting (Bohleber, 2010). Gaps are often filled in utilizing the body as conduit of the narrative. It remains incumbent upon both patient and analyst in the analytic dyad to translate the body's messages into thought.

Bion, following Freud, explored the conditions and experiences that are necessary for the development of an apparatus for thinking thoughts, which involves linking sense impressions and affects with concepts that have meaning and language that can be used for thought and communication (Stevens, 2009, pp. 522–523). Bion's idea of the caesura, in particular, is an interesting and a wide-ranging concept that generalizes to all aspects of the personality, real and imagined. The caesura theoretically constitutes a separating contact-barrier that, with its "selective permeability", allows for the controlled passage of psychic elements back and forth between consciousness and the unconscious, also allowing for connections and integration of such paradoxical elements as past and present, inside and outside, reality and fantasy, primitive sensory elements and symbolic functioning (Grotstein, 2007, pp. 257–258).

Inherent in Bion's concept of caesura is the idea of transformation by way of differentiation. Such transformation allows for the ability to move easily between the world of primitive, sensory experience and the world of symbolic thought (Anderson, 2014). Patients who cannot easily do this are deemed "concrete", and often have traumatic early histories (Frosch, 2012). The term "caesura", then, may be used to elucidate the humanizing function of reverie which Bion considered vital for psychic growth (Bion, 1977/1989; Anderson, 2014).

In terms of Bion's viewpoint, failure of the reverie function leads to the collapse of the caesura, a state of dedifferentiation where rage is unbounded and one can become "lost in space." When there is "violence at the caesura" such as trauma, there is a reversion to a concrete way of operating (Anderson, 2014). This idea seems very reminiscent of Freud's discussion of the "stimulus barrier", that protective filter for physiologic and psychological stimuli that can be penetrated by traumatic events. Freud's view of the nature of the traumatic neurosis was discussed in *Beyond the Pleasure Principle* (1920) along with the compulsion to repeat. According to Freud, a disturbance arises when the ego is totally unprepared for a "traumatizing" event of an external kind. The stimulus barrier breaks down and the ego is overwhelmed with an anxiety that cannot be mastered at the time.

The cumulative trauma inherent in the deficits in the mother–infant dyad in Ms. D's early history, as well as the secondary enuresis and the invasive urological examinations and treatment that followed, all can be understood in terms of "violence at the caesura". The natural flow of emotionality, as well as the differentiation between inside and outside, was compromised.

In order to defend against such intrapsychic violence, Ms. D has often been profoundly resistant to change within and without. Until recently she did not feel safe enough to utilize the function of reverie, to freely associate. In some ways, neither did I. Analytic "playing" in a transitional space had been difficult to achieve and maintain on an ongoing basis. According to Anderson and others, concrete experience, in a patient such as Ms. D, often resides as embodied memory consisting of unmetabolized sensory elements that are enacted through the body (Anderson, 2014; Lemma, 2015).

For Ms. D, moving from an unknowable, undifferentiated reality into a mental space where "attentiveness, receptivity, tolerance, and patience" could give "shape and depth" to her experience (Anderson, 2014) has been a slow, painstaking process. She has needed to develop a greater ability to tolerate and bridge contradictory mental states. I have come to understand that the development of this capacity throughout her treatment has been continuously subject to a kind of violence from within, due to unprocessed memories of the early trauma that worked as a constant pull toward dedifferentiation. This did not allow Ms. D to fully develop a mature internal structure that would allow for greater tolerance for emotional pain and a full-on capacity for reflective thought.

As noted, the oscillation between Ms. D's unbearable desire for me (the heightened state of arousal) and her stultifying need for distance often rendered her unreachable. This was especially true whenever I mentioned a topic that was deemed "off limits" (such as her father's death). At these moments Ms. D would stiffen her body and her face would simultaneously reflect fear, physical pain and loathing—and she would often squeeze her legs together. As I said, Ms. D would act as though I were performing an overstimulating, torturous act on her—much like her mother's simultaneous intrusiveness and emotional "deadness"—as well as the pediatrician's clinically cold vaginal examinations.

Bach (2002a), in his discussion of sadomasochism, emphasized the cumulative traumatic experience inherent in a dysfunctional mother–infant dyad where there is a lack of parental attunement. It is speculated that ongoing emotional neglect of this nature is experienced by the child as a series of betrayals that undermine the development of a solid sense of self and other. The child fights against deep attachment to someone so emotionally distant and/or unpredictable and feels constantly enraged and overwhelmed. Typically, the rage cannot be expressed and the child ends by shaming and blaming herself for not being able to reach the mother whom she has idealized to protect her from her aggression.

Ms. D was (and is) enraged at her mother, but dared not express that rage. Indeed, she was overwhelmed by it and the anxiety surrounding it. Her mother did not adequately protect her and did not allow her any freedom. This was traumatizing. Consequently Ms. D had trouble in developing her own sense of agency. As Bach further points out,

> such sadomasochistic dyads are a closely coupled system without autonomy for either caretaker or child, who have indeed both become each other's slaves. A normal dyad is loosely coupled, so that while each partner can experience togetherness, he can also experience moments of aloneness, autonomy, and effectance. (2002a)

Furthermore, the closed union of the sadomasochistic dyad not only impedes autonomy but it also excludes the oedipal third, so that illusory aspects are maintained at the expense of an entry into reality: the real, triadic, oedipal world (Green, 2004). Since Ms. D could not express her hatred to her mother and did not obtain any pleasure from her, her rage seems to have become sexualized and displaced elsewhere in "a perverted demand for love". This was furthered by the very real absence of Ms. D's father, who worked a lot (even on weekends) and therefore did not offer Ms. D a good enough link to the real world. One may speculate that Ms. D's enuresis, though congenitally driven, may have, secondarily, become a "perverted demand for love", where both losing control and forcing control of the bladder may have been exciting as well as frightening. All of this became revivified and enacted within our analytic dyad.

According to Maxine Anderson (2014, p. 342), "Ordinary mothering usually secures [the] potential for change within the baby but if there is failure of this attentiveness, especially in the early stages of emotional unfolding, the vulnerable self may feel exposed once again to the de-differentiating sweep back into the inchoate, that impersonal real"—in other words, that "violence at the caesura".

Such exposure to these unprocessed elements (beta elements, in Bionion terms) can be experienced as violently destabilizing. Anderson notes that:

> Without the protective shield of mother's mind the vulnerable ego feels exposed to the brutality of unfiltered reality. One defensive response to this overwhelm may be to erect a wall, to rigidify the potential dialectic into frozen polarized, non-communicating positions: instead of a dialectical interchange absolute differences appear, and polar opposites and convictions freeze into place. (Anderson, 2014, p. 342)

It has become clearer to me and to Ms. D that her mother (who was chronically depressed, narcissistic and incapable of a secure form of mothering) could not adequately shield Ms. D from such "unfiltered reality". This, perhaps, was especially true during Ms. D's infancy and early childhood. Instead, mother intruded upon Ms. D in ways that felt violently assaultive and Ms. D, in turn, was flooded with a primitive annihilation anxiety. As a consequence, Ms. D developed splits within her psyche in order to cope. The assaultive nature of this overwhelming pressure of reality was repeated later in Ms. D's childhood during the pediatrician's probing of Ms. D's vagina while performing intrusive examinations of her bladder. Under these circumstances she felt horribly alone and unprotected.

In our sessions, by labeling my own thoughts and feelings as well as by noticing and commenting on Ms. D's facial expressions and body movements, I was able to help Ms. D transcend what seemed to be a fixed immovable gap within her, where her body was the only recourse for communication. This was a "humanizing" experience for her, and in some way my observations could be likened to a mother responding to and commenting on her infant's smiles and grimaces—the body language inherent in the normal dialogue between mother and baby. My comments, I believe, created a bridge for Ms. D that helped foster a transformation in her inner world that allowed her to integrate dissociated, split-off parts.

Ms. D's subsequent willingness to utilize the couch has been an interesting and important move forward, and we both view it as a significant achievement. However, it has not gone unnoticed that it is also, perhaps, a defense against my reading her facial expressions. We are both aware of this, and so Ms. D herself came up with the solution of my moving my chair in such a way that I could still see her face, although she could only see my feet. "Seeing your feet is enough for me, now—at least most of the time," she recently said. It seems a good compromise.

References

Anderson, M.K. (2014). Violence at the caesura. *Canadian Journal of Psychoanalysis*, 22: 339–349.

Bach, S. (2002a). Sadomasochism in clinical practice and everyday life. *Journal of Clinical Psychoanalysis*, 11(2): 225–235.

Bach, S. (2002b). A mind of one's own: Some observations on disorders of thinking. *Symbolization and Desymbolization: Essays in Honor of Norbert Freedman*, Lasky, R. (ed.). New York: Other Press.

Bach, S. (2011). Chimeras: Immunity, interpenetration, and the true self. *Psychoanalytic Review*, 98(1): 39–56.

Bion, W.R. (1959). Attacks on linking. *International Journal of Psycho-Analysis*, 40: 308–315.

Bion, W.R. (1977/1989). *Caesura, in Two Papers: The Grid and Caesura*. London: Karnac.

Bohleber, W. (2010). *Destructiveness, Intersubjectivity and Trauma: The Identity Crisis of Modern Psychoanalysis*. London: Karnac.

Davies, J.M. (2004). Whose bad objects are we anyway? Repetition and our elusive love affair. *Psychoanalytic Dialogues*, 14: 711–732.

Ellman, P. & Goodman, N. (2012). Enactment: Opportunity for symbolising trauma. *Absolute Truth and Unbearable Psychic Pain: Psychoanalytic Perspectives on Concrete Experience*, A. Frosch (ed.). London: Karnac, 57–72.

Fonagy, P. & Target, M. (1998). Mentalization and the changing aims of child psychoanalysis. *Psychoanalytic Dialogues*, 8(1): 87–114.

Freud, S. (1920). Beyond the pleasure principle. *Standard Edition 18*: 1–64.

Frosch, A., ed. (2012). *Absolute Truth and Unbearable Psychic Pain: Psychoanalytic Perspectives on Concrete Experience*. London: Karnac.

Green, A. (2004). Thirdness and psychoanalytic concepts. *Psychoanalytic Quarterly*, 73: 99–135.

Grotstein, J.S. (2007). *A Beam of Intense Darkness: Wilfred Bion's Legacy to Psychoanalysis*. London: Karnac.

Lemma, A. (2015). *Minding the Body: The Body in Psychoanalysis and Beyond*. New York: Routledge.

Leuzinger-Bohleber, M. (2008). Biographical truths and their clinical consequences: Understanding "embodied memories" in a third psychoanalysis with a traumatized patient recovered from severe poliomyelitis. *International Journal of Psychoanalysis*, 89(6): 1165–1187.

Leuzinger-Bohleber, M. & Pfeifer, R. (2002). Remembering a depressive primary object. *International Journal of Psychoanalysis*, 83(1): 3–33.

Rifkin, M. (2013). Toxic impasse: Loss and recovery of the analyst's mind, *Round Robin: APA Section 1 Newsletter*, 18(1): 1–7.

Stevens, V. (2009). *Bion, Klein, and Freud*. S.J. Ellman, *When Theories Touch: A Historical and Theoretical Integration of Psychoanalytic Thought: A Historical and Theoretical Integration of Psychoanalytic Thought*. London: Karnac, 521–540.

Part III

Political catastrophes

Chapter 9

Trauma and the fate of nations

Robert L. Pyles

The fate of nations and individuals is often shaped by devastating trauma. Such events are frequently experienced by both, with an overwhelming and long-lasting sense of humiliation and helplessness. Both the experience of the events and the subsequent attempts to cope become integrated in the national and personal character.[1]

On December 7, 1941, with no declaration of war, Japanese planes attacked Pearl Harbor, devastating the US Pacific Fleet. In his address to the people of the United States, President Franklin D. Roosevelt denounced the "sneak" attack as "a day which will live in infamy."

For the Japanese, the twin goals of their action were to destroy American military capability in the Pacific, but mainly, through the sudden and overwhelming force of the assault, to break the will of the American people. The result was hardly what the Japanese had intended. Even Fleet Commander Nagumo, realizing they had missed the American aircraft carriers, commented, "I fear that all we have accomplished is to awaken a sleeping giant, and fill him with a terrible resolve."

In the history of any nation, there are a relatively few watershed events that define a people and a national character. For the United States, in addition to Pearl Harbor, those would be the Revolution in 1776 and the subsequent establishment of the Constitution, the Civil War (1861–1865), which produced a greater loss of life than all other US wars combined, and Pearl Harbor.

And then there was September 11, 2001.

The horrific attacks on the World Trade Center and the Pentagon in Washington, DC, bear superficial similarities to the attack on Pearl Harbor. Both came without warning and with extreme violence, both resulted in massive loss of life, and both stunned the nation. But there the comparison stops.

The Japanese attack was intended to coincide with a formal declaration of war. The Japanese government felt some constraint to operate within the rules of warfare recognized by civilized nations. The assault was strictly aimed at military personnel and equipment. The goal was professionally political and strategic. Oddly, as shocking as it was, it didn't feel personal; nor did it feel motivated by hatred.

The terrorist attacks, by contrast, occurred with unmitigated and deliberate savagery, against a completely civilian population. Rather than being similar to Pearl Harbor, these attacks belong on the list with Bosnia, the Holocaust and Cambodia. These are crimes of "ethnic cleansing". The motivation is racial hatred. The goal is genocide—or to paralyze a people.

In the aftermath of the attacks, as people recovered from the initial shock, the most common bewildered questions were "Why do they hate us so much?" and "How could anyone kill so many innocent people?" These are vital questions on which political leaders, psychoanalysts and others must work together to answer.

What psychological forces must operate to create a mind set in which individuals or groups become capable of forsaking their basic humanity and perpetrating mass slaughter? There is no question that much of the answer must lie in the understanding of group dynamics. In 1921, in his groundbreaking work "Group Psychology and the Analysis of the Ego", Sigmund Freud wrote about the necessary factors for the cohesiveness of a group. In his view, it required a central organizing idea or belief system, a charismatic leader, or both. Freud and many others have pointed out that membership in a group, particularly one that requires relatively unquestioning allegiance, depends upon a suspension of critical judgment on the part of the adherents. The individual sense of personal identity becomes fused with that of the group.

Thus membership in a group with a strong central belief system requires setting aside the ordinary ability of the ego to assess what might be thought of as rational reality. In psychoanalytic terms, this amounts to a regression to the more primitive ego mechanisms—splitting, projection, denial and distortion. In this kind of group, which Bion (1961) would have called a "basic needs group", paranoia and isolationism become paramount. The primary function of the group becomes the need to distinguish between "me and not-me"; that is, those who are like me (my group) and those who are not like me (everyone else). The character functioning of the group becomes intensely narcissistic.

Religious or faith-based groups represent a particular aspect of group dynamics. Ordinarily, these are not problematic because, while each religion has its own belief system, the group has not lost its connection and sense of identification with the rest of humanity. The five major religions of Christianity, Judaism, Buddhism, Hinduism and Islam all have specific doctrines of peace and tolerance of other religions.

Fundamentalist religious groups, such as Al-Qaeda, are another matter altogether. Ironically, their belief systems have much more in common with each other than with the parent religion of which they are a part. They invariably seek to return to a glorious past, and see the present as corrupt and obscene. (This current effort seems to have at its root a wish to turn the clock back 1000 years, to the great days of Muslim hegemony.) They have the sense that their cultural or national group has been betrayed and humiliated, and they seek to reclaim their honor by humiliating others. They feel economically and politically impotent.

In World War II, 6 million Jews, and possibly 50 million others, died. In Bosnia, perhaps 50,000. It can happen again. And again. This is the most clear and present danger. An unchecked feeling of personal or group defectiveness, essentially a narcissistic regression, leads directly to the rationalized slaughter of the "other".

These groups are marked by the most primitive of ego mechanisms. Hatred and suspicion of others, intolerance, exclusiveness, isolation and blind adherence to their own belief system as the one true faith are their hallmarks. The gate of independent reasoning is closed. In the individual, we would call this psychotic, a profoundly narcissistic character organization, but there are no comparable terms in group dynamics. There is a grandiose sense of fusion with God, a certainty that the will of God is being carried out. As we have seen throughout human history, killing for political reasons can be bad enough, but killing for the will of God carries with it unlimited savagery.

This brings us to the most essential element that underlies massacre—the need to dehumanize the other. I first encountered this phenomenon when I was a Lt. Commander in the US Navy during Viet Nam. Serving as a psychiatrist, it was part of my duty to treat Marines just two days out of the combat line. Many of these young men, mostly teenagers or in their early twenties, had seen frequent combat, and had often seen their friends and comrades die or be mangled in horrible ways. They described a nightmare situation—jungle, an unseen enemy, death constantly lurking. Anyone, an elderly villager, a nine-year old boy, could and would carry a hidden grenade.

To cope, many of these young soldiers came to see all Vietnamese as "gooks", "slants", "dinks". And, as such, they became easier to kill. These boys could not kill a Vietnamese teenager who might be like themselves, or their younger brother. But they could kill a "gook". Or lay down a curtain of fire on a village and ask questions later. It didn't happen often. But it happened. And sometimes they felt guilt—and sometimes they didn't.

A diagnosis of a major aspect of the problem should also suggest an approach to a solution. Such a belief system as the terrorists advocate is based on splitting, the distinction between the grandiose self and the denigrated self. This can only flourish to the extent that the people of Islam are kept in isolation and ignorance. If this is true, then inclusion, dialogue and mutual exchange must be the long-term goals. This would be policy based on the most sound of political, psychological and social goals. It is instructive to see what it is that our self-professed enemies, the fundamentalist leadership, most fear, and that is clearly the inclusion and influence of other cultures. This would mean the end to the isolation of their people, and the end of fundamentalism. As the Prophet predicted, Islam would be united into the world community.

Unfortunately, short-term solutions are much more clouded. It is likely that the last thing that the hard-core fundamentalists would welcome is open dialogue. And who would doubt that the Bin Ladens of the world and their followers would kill us all if they had the means. Therefore, counterforce, until more moderate governments can be assembled, seems inevitable. Nonetheless, mutual cultural education, economic aid and interchange with the Muslim people and those of all faiths must remain our most potent weapon.

Targets of terrorism

People everywhere have mixed feelings; but there is a steely resolve to do whatever is necessary to bring terrorism to heel, and to punish those individuals and countries responsible for this modern version of a biblical scourge. But there is also widespread anxiety. The most ordinary things seem dangerous—taking a trip, opening the mail, etc. This raises the question: How can the roots of terrorism, the effect on the victim or victim group, be understood psychologically?

The goal of terrorism is to strike at one of the most basic elements of the human psyche, the sense of safety. Terrorism seeks to create the impression that there is no safe place, nowhere to hide. Disaster may strike from anywhere. People, places or things which were once taken for granted can now become instruments of destruction. A letter can kill. The renter down the hall becomes a murderous hijacker. A commercial plane becomes a deadly missile.

Television and the media have greatly augmented the effect of terrorist activities. Who will ever be able to erase from their consciousness the sight of airliners hitting the World Trade Center Towers; or the Towers, crumbling, one after another, like children's toys; or the daily newspaper reports of the latest anthrax scare. Our own freedoms have become the terrorists' most potent weapons.

In the first instance, the death of thousands strikes violently and without warning. The images are replayed 1000 times. In the second, death is silent and insidious, and may come unseen, anywhere and anytime. Do I dare to fly? Is the train safer? But there's no security check on the train! Is that white substance baby powder, or could it be anthrax? How do we know they don't have access to nuclear devices or smallpox? Like a panic attack, the fear of a possible terrorist attack becomes a far more potent weapon than the few actual attacks. Once this state of mind is achieved in a populace, the terrorists' work is done. All it takes are a few unpredictable incidents here or there to keep it going.

Hollywood seems intuitively to have long understood the essence of fear as described by Freud in his 1919 paper "The Uncanny". Freud used the word *heimlich*, which in German means "homelike" or "pertaining to the hearth", the essence of safety and warm security. But a slight alteration in the word, *unheimlich*, turns it into the opposite, and it comes to mean something that is strange or frightening. As he puts it, "uncanny is that class of frightening which leads back to what is known of old and long familiar." Freud goes on to point out that what is the most fear-inducing, what truly inspires terror, is not what is totally alien and different, but that which seems familiar but strangely altered.

Movies like *The Invasion of the Body Snatchers*, in which trusted friends and relatives turn out to be blood-hungry invaders from space, make effective use of this primal fear. Or *Psycho*, where the sweet adolescent boy is in fact a murderous schizophrenic, and a relaxing shower becomes a death-trap. An early example is Count Dracula, a monster in human form, who drains the life of all who cross his path.

The power of terrorism rests in its ability to undermine our beliefs that we can determine what is safe and what is not. Terrorists seek to convince us that we can no longer rely on what we thought was real. Everything is designed to shake our faith in the reality assumptions by which we live our lives.

Terrorists in general, but these in particular, make it clear that, although they seem human and look human, they are bound by no human convention. There are no laws or rules that they are not eager to violate. Even the most basic of human instincts, that of self-preservation, has no meaning. Bin Laden commented that while Bush sought life, he sought death. What could be a more fundamental denial of all that we hold dear?

The universal human wish to protect the innocent and helpless, like women and children, does not hold. There is no act so merciless that they will not commit it. Random murder is the norm. Mass destruction is the goal.

This tactic is deliberate, though not necessarily conscious, and the goal is to paralyze the enemy by a fear so profound and primitive that resistance will be impossible.

So what can be done to combat such a different and subversive enemy? Part of the problem is our own denial. We don't want to accept that people can behave with such mindless hatred. We invent euphemisms to cover up what we don't want to see. Such attacks become "work-place violence" or "man-caused disasters".

But we must face up to the reality, difficult as it is. We need to recognize that this is essentially a fascist enemy, dressed in different clothes, more than a religious one, as old as mankind itself. The beginning of any fascist movement has relatively few fanatically devoted followers. Such a movement is a danger not only to the US and Israel, but also to the whole civilized world because the very tenets of civilization are being attacked. The need to establish a global antiterrorism network, with both military and intelligence capabilities, is paramount.

What can we do to protect our personal psychological well-being? Just as our sense of reality can be used against us, it is also our main ally. The sense of reality is the precise target of terrorism. The terrorists are few in number. They are human and vulnerable. We have massive advantages in numbers and resources, and they know that. Security and health measures are, and have been, rapidly put into place. We have gotten a wake-up call, and we are responding.

Our global and personal character is being tested. Our children are looking to us for guidance and direction. We would do well to remember the words of President Roosevelt after Pearl Harbor, as he rallied our nation and the world to the cause: "The only thing we have to fear is fear itself."

It would be ironic and fitting if the ultimate effect of September 11 were to result in the greater understanding between Islam and the rest of the world. The achievement of this mutual understanding and openness would spell the death of terrorism and hatred, and would result in the triumph of the human spirit, in both people and nations.

Note

1 An earlier version of this chapter was presented at the CIPA/NAPsaC Clinical Conference on Trauma, Destruction and Transformative Potential in New York City, May 2014.

References

Bion, W.R. (1961). *Experiences in Groups.* London: Tavistock.

Freud, S. (1919). The uncanny. *Standard Edition 17*: 217–256. London: Hogarth Press.

Freud, S. (1921). Group psychology and the analysis of the ego. *Standard Edition 18.* London: Hogarth Press.

Chapter 10

Learning to live with ghosts

Linking trauma to an intergenerational collective past

Susan S. Berger

Psychoanalytic literature and recent biological research (Zaiden et al., 2013; Gainsler-Salomon, 2014) as well as life and clinical experience undeniably point to the fact that intergenerational transmission of trauma is both widespread and insidious. It operates on all levels, within the most personal and intimate relationships, as well as between and within nations. It affects groups that are pitted against each other and competing for resources; and it influences institutions, including psychoanalytic institutes and organizations. As psychoanalysts, we operate on the premise that the more we are able to understand the origins and mechanisms of trauma's transmission, the more we can mitigate its self-perpetuating power. We are painfully privy to both the content and process of its destructive force, but also privileged to be in the position to intervene in order to dilute its effect and turn that force against itself. By developing an awareness of the full breadth and depth of intergenerational trauma, we help not only our patients but can also strengthen our impact on the organizations and institutions we are a part of.

Many notable authors have affirmed the frequent, intense and parallel reliving of parental trauma in offspring, particularly, though not exclusively, among Holocaust survivor families (Fraiberg et al., 1975; Bergmann & Jucovy, 1982; Kestenberg, 1980; 1993; Laub, 1998; Auerhahn & Laub, 1998; Fromm, 2011; Charles, 2012). In "Whose Trauma Is It Anyway? Towards Furthering Our Understanding of Its Intergenerational Transmission" (Berger, 2014), I provided some case examples of how closely the particular experience of the parents was relived in the second generation of Holocaust survivors. In that paper I suggest utilizing Bion's theory of group dynamics (1961) in looking at how family dynamics affect intrapsychic development. More specifically, Bion's concept of the "work group" and its functioning in terms of task, authority, roles and boundary can serve as a kind of scaffolding that links the past to the present, as well as the individual to the group, in a broad range of situations and psychological dilemmas. This multi-layered and theoretically interwoven approach to the individual, the family and, even further, to a range of identity groups struggling with the effects of collective trauma can enrich clinical work and increase its effectiveness. While the clinical examples I used to demonstrate the usefulness of this approach were based on the collective trauma of the Holocaust, I maintain that it can apply to those whose family history includes slavery and racism, war-related and other violence, homophobic assaults, and many other forms of collective and intergenerational trauma.

While certainly not all trauma is derived from some form of intergenerational experience, once trauma occurs, there's no doubt that it has the potential to reverberate, with the original source becoming lost to conscious memory. Social environment most certainly has an important role to play in all trauma, and its underlying and critical influence is generally acknowledged in the healing process. Collective/group trauma almost always seems to have an intergenerational component, both in terms of its origins and its sustainability. Directly addressing and/or acknowledging greater social and historical context is therefore within the purview of clinical work, providing a basis in reality that has greater integrity than limiting its scope to the individual, the family and parent–child relationships.

Previously, I attempted to address some complex and multi-level factors involved in how terror of an external threat can be internalized (Berger, 2014). I made a case for incorporating concepts from group relations and systems-psychoanalytic thinking to help bridge our understanding of the links between group experience and individual, intrapsychic experience.

Thinking about family functioning within a systemic frame in working individually with an adult, whether during the course of reconstruction or when focusing on the present, can be an important asset to understanding a patient's experience. Patterns that emerge in the transference also provide important information regarding the patient's role within relationships, how he or she relates to authority, and the ability to discern and maintain boundaries. These qualities refer directly to Bion's theory of group anxieties and the work group further elucidated by others working within a socio-analytic and systems-psychoanalytic framework (Green & Molenkamp, 2005; White, 2002).

Referring to group historical, as well as current, experience does not detract from exploring and working with the deepest intrapsychic processes and fantasies. In fact, it is my experience that it broadens and strengthens the frame, freeing the patient and analyst to explore and work through what are often powerful formative and transformative internal processes. Making these links explicit also enables the patient to better utilize the insights gained in the consulting room in other domains.

Until now, more easily identifiable intergenerational issues, such as the Holocaust and child or domestic abuse, have been a frequent focus in the exploration of intergenerational trauma in the psychoanalytic literature. By using a case example of someone with a history of other collective trauma, in addition to the Holocaust, I hope to demonstrate the importance and usefulness of expanding our clinical thinking about the transmission of trauma intergenerationally to include a significantly greater percentage of our patients.

Ariel was referred at age 6 for her oppositional stance towards learning. Also of concern to her teachers and parents was a tendency to talk about people and events that were either blatantly or later discovered to be imaginary. These tall tales often included nonexistent family members, and focused on major milestones such as a wedding or birth of a child, and also on deaths. She also often made statements that reflected her wishes as if they were a reality. A thorough psycho-educational evaluation ruled out neurologically based learning issues. Developmental history includes an easy temperament as a baby and no significant or unusual traumatic events during her early development.

In the first few months of treatment, Ariel's sessions took on a ritualistic format. We began by playing a war-genre board game (Stratego), popular among 9- to 12-year-old boys, but not typically of interest to a girl her age. We played the game very loosely in terms of adherence to the rules, in part because at 6 she wasn't yet able to fully comprehend the rules and complexities of different strategies, but mainly because the necessary and only important factor for her was that she won the war. It was only after her experience of victory that Ariel was free to engage in activities that were more usual for girls her age. Most frequently, she would create drawings that almost always included the names of family members. She also often drew pictures of food.

Another component of our sessions in the first few months was her repetitive questioning of how long she'd be coming in to see me. At first this questioning was done with an oppositional tone, as if it was something she'd rather not continue; but with time and a greater sense of attachment, her questioning was more clearly an outgrowth of anxiety. She asked for reassurance that we'd meet through the coming school year, and possibly next year, too. She told her mother that she didn't understand why she resisted coming to see me, because she really enjoyed it.

While the content of sessions is certainly multiply determined, I have considered that her great-grandfather (an active part of her life) surviving the Holocaust as a child as a relevant factor in understanding the dynamics of the case. While it was never appropriate to make any Holocaust-related interpretations in my work with this girl, it was certainly addressed in my work with her parents. Her mother, who had a special bond with her Holocaust-survivor grandparent, for the very first time became aware of the impact of her grandfather's experience on family dynamics, formative experiences and often overwhelming anxiety. Addressing this directly in the parent sessions had an immediate positive impact on the parents' marriage and the mother's emotional availability to her children.

There are also cases in which intergenerational transmission of trauma emerges less blatantly. Peter, an analysand originally from an Eastern European country with a history of domination by and violent conflict with a neighboring nation, has suffered from various anxiety-related symptoms—many of which are socially related—as well as bouts of depression, beginning in childhood, according to his recollection. His anxiety was intensified by a health-related traumatic event a few years ago: It was in the aftermath of this event that he developed a pervasive feeling of having been violated in some way, which initially brought him into treatment. The degree of Peter's social anxiety is particularly notable given his success in a field in which interpersonal skills are critical.

While Peter grew up in what was in many ways a typical middle-class family, there were several factors in his own history of traumas that clearly played an important role in his symptoms, and his reaction to the more recent experience. Peter had two surgeries at ages 6 and 7, one a circumcision (the medical reason for this is not completely clear to him) and the other to correct a urethral blockage not long after the circumcision (his fantasy was that it was the result of the circumcision). Additionally, he experienced a traumatic hospitalization at age 9 because of an infected laceration: He was placed in an adult ward with men whose injuries and state of health were particularly gruesome.

The incident was especially revealing of his relationship with his father. Peter was injured when he slipped and fell as he excitedly went to greet him arriving home from work. Despite being a loving and responsible parent, Peter's father strongly disapproved of expressions of such excitement and other forms of emotionality in his son (though not his daughter), and the injury and subsequent horrifying experiences were internalized as the inevitable result of what was transmitted to Peter as an "overly" emotional reaction and "less masculine" inner experience.

As our work evolved, sessions centered on the traumas in his history as well as other early experiences, family dynamics, neurotic conflicts and defensive patterns of withdrawal and obsessive interpersonal strategizing, which initially included planning what he would talk about in his sessions. However, Peter's engagement in his treatment seemed also to be significantly enhanced by pointing to links between his emotional experience and factors often not addressed in psychoanalysis, at least as reported in case discussions. More specifically, at times I made interpretations connecting his internal experience with systems and organizational components of his work environment, as well as aspects of his national identity and socio-cultural history as the session material presented seemed to reflect them.

For example, in discussing Peter's father's lack of tolerance of his young son's expressions of excitement and overall intense emotional temperament, I wondered if part of what was affecting the father was a fear that Peter would become stereotyped as impulsive and potentially dangerous to others. I also wondered if his father feared he would possibly be attracted to what was then a violent nationalistic movement. In understanding his father and his overly rigid protective impulse towards Peter, and Peter's reactions to it, oedipal conflicts have certainly been brought to light. However, the impact of stories of young men being imprisoned, or worse, as a result of expressions of national pride were also given some attention in understanding the fuller picture of the social environment. These factors were considered as possibly having a role in his struggle with the conflicts and inhibitions interfering with his performance at work, as well as overall pleasure and satisfaction in life.

Keeping the socio-historical and cultural factors in mind, and at times including them in my comments and interpretations to the patient, played a role, I believe—based on the clinical material that followed—in deepening the work. These factors could be understood as supporting the containing function of the analytic frame, as the psychic space is developed to explore psychic realities. Realities of time and place frame not only our experience but also our identity. The analyst's interest in learning more about these factors not only serves as a reinforcement of the containing function of analytic work, especially during the earlier phases of treatment; it can also be experienced by the patient as an invitation to be a more active participant in the development and maintenance of the work.

Within analytic literature (Blum, 1986; 1987; Freud, 1936/1966), turning passive into active with regard to trauma is ubiquitous and, clinically, an undeniably powerful and central force in its amelioration. While turning passive into active refers to identification with the aggressor, it isn't limited to that. Understanding the roots as well as the complexities of victimization can help free the patient from self-blame and feelings of powerlessness. The experience of being an active participant in the development and maintenance of analytic work is therefore also critical in supporting the ability to synthesize and internalize new experiences generated both in and outside the analytic situation.

In other words, keeping the external realities of time and place in mind, in addition to other psychic realities unfolding within the analytic process, can lessen the narcissistic wounds inherent in the development of emotional symptomatology (Oliner, 1966; Van der Kolk et al., 1966). The egocentricity of a child's perspective makes a defense that evolves into a symptom serve as proof of inadequacy and even self-destructive tendencies. Understanding the necessity of these defenses in response to traumatic historical circumstances and their reverberations can help challenge and eventually ameliorate this belief or inner fantasy, thus relieving the underlying experience and perpetuation of victimization. This includes working not only with analysands, but also the parents of child and adolescent patients, as demonstrated in Ariel's case. The critical support of parents in their containing role for their children's anxieties necessitates this approach. Additionally, as with analysands, pointing to socio-cultural and historical factors can also lessen the inherent narcissistic vulnerability in parenting. For example, for Peter, highly educated and well-read, there already was an awareness of links among his cultural identity, sense of self and narcissistic vulnerabilities. He referred in his treatment to Nelson Mandela and Mahatma Gandhi as idealized figures, and had fantasies in his youth of being a war correspondent. Interpersonally, he thought of himself as a wizard behind a curtain rather than fully engaging with others.

Six-year-old Ariel often refers to her cultural and (multi)religious heritage in sessions, as well as expressing curiosity about mine. The clinician's entrance into this domain of the patient's experience in a self-aware, multi-dimensional and open manner can fundamentally strengthen the alliance and further the exploratory and integrative work of treatment.

Thinking about the organizational functioning of a family, issues that arise in the workplace or other group situations and issues related to identity can all serve as a link between the socio-cultural and the intra-psychic. Peter's father's compliant attitude towards authority and active attempts to suppress his son's emotional expression have many determinants. It also became an important area of exploration as Peter struggled to increase his capacity to compete and fully utilize his talents and capabilities in the workplace. While Peter's exceptional analytical skills and steadfast work ethic enabled him to advance professionally, he frequently had to surmount an almost paralyzing anxiety. This resulted in significantly slowing the pace of his advancement by what was ultimately understood as obstacles arising from intra-psychic factors.

Exploration of the many layers of these intra-psychic factors was, of course, dictated by the material that Peter brought into his sessions. Most often on the surface, and experienced as most urgent during the course of his analysis in the earlier stages, was Peter's workplace experience. The socio-analytic and systems-psychoanalytic conceptual framework has enriched how I listen as well as comment on the material presented. The centrality of the unconscious, as well as a multi-faceted and complex approach to relationships and psychic development, enables socio-analytic or systems-psychoanalytic thinking to be applicable to psychoanalytic treatment.

Listening for the role that Peter repeatedly took on in his work and in relationship to authority, such as an exaggerated caretaker role with his supervisor, led to an exploration of his role within his family and, most particularly, with his parents. It deepened into explorations related to oedipal issues as one of the inhibitors of competition and perceived expressions of aggression in the workplace, as well as linking them to issues of dependency and separation, including within the transference. These many layers were traversed over the course of the analysis as the various parts of his experience and identity were integrated and synthesized into a more cohesive whole.

Similarly, the awareness of the many layers and complex interweaving of the intra-psychic elements of his dilemma opened a pathway to addressing the inclusion of intergenerational transmission of trauma. In talking about his decision to attend graduate school in the US, Peter stated that "there was nothing holding" him in his country of origin. He also described deciding against attending a graduate school in the neighboring country with which there was a history of domination and violent conflict, even though it was closer geographically. He feared, with some justification, that he would always be looked upon suspiciously and negatively as a result of his national identity, and that this would ultimately limit his potential for professional success and his quality of life socially.

The influence of the history of national conflict on Peter's personal experience as reflected in the session material enabled me to make the link between his father's anxiety about being, as well as raising a son who might be "hot-headed" and "overly-aggressive", and his own deeply embedded conflicts and inhibitions. The very strong emphasis on work and achievement, including in athletics, to the exclusion of emotional expression was linked to the father's wishes and needs for power and safety in the world and in their relationship. Certainly, issues of castration anxiety as experienced because of his surgeries, and the way they were handled by his parents and medical personnel, were influenced in many ways by the culture. (Both parents were brought up in religious homes.) Anxieties about sexuality were intensified not only by a strong sense of the forbidden, but also traumas associated with a history of violent oppression by a more powerful nation. The history of poverty and hunger, as well as the sexual exploitation by those in power, also served as a powerful backdrop to the family's functioning and Peter's individual development.

Keeping these collective traumas in mind, I believe, enables the clinician to maintain a focus on the patient's experience rather than the pathology and maladaptive characteristics of the symptomatology. For example, when thinking about feeling the lack of "holding" Peter experienced, one might legitimately wonder about the quality of object relations or attachment in the family. However, the tensions and conflicts described by Peter over the course of his treatment strongly suggested a connection to cultural patterns and expectation of emigration often related to economic opportunities. Almost all of his mother's many siblings have resided in foreign countries since young adulthood. Emotional turmoil and instability in family life, despite the experience of close ties, was a fact of life with repercussions—marital strife resulting in divorce occurred frequently within the extended family. Additionally, Peter's mother had been very close to a sibling who tragically committed suicide after struggling with alcoholism for many years, leaving behind an estranged wife and children. This traumatic loss, and the history of her brother's emotional struggles, greatly affected her parenting. Peter's experience of the loss of this uncle for his mother and grandparents, and the resulting burden of responsibility for repair of this family trauma, had been profound as it emerged in the analysis. As in the cases of children of Holocaust survivors (Berger 2014; Bergmann & Jucovy, 1982; Faimberg 1988, Kestenberg, 1980; 1993; Laub, 1998; Auerhahn & Laub, 1998), there has been a significant loss of a sense of self in this process of repair, which has hampered Peter's sense of agency and regulation of self-esteem and, therefore, profoundly contributed to his overall anxiety and bouts of depression.

The intense experience of loss of an extended family member, as well as many other experiences—including a very close relationship with his maternal grandparents—speaks to the strength of family bonds. This in turn speaks to the emotional upheaval of the geographical dispersion of the family. As in the case of the Holocaust families described in an earlier paper (Berger, 2014), thinking about the family as a work group, based on Bion's theoretical framework, has been useful. Given the socio-economic and political history in Peter's background, the traumatic losses can be viewed as personal, familial and collective/cultural.

Keeping Peter's experience of himself in relation to the family group, with regard to the experience of this uncle's suicide and how the information was relayed, or not, in Peter's case, presented a particularly poignant moment in the analysis. Upon discovering that his uncle's death was, in fact, a suicide and not the result of an accident, and that he was the only one—including cousins his age—who didn't know this, he recalled how profoundly disturbing this was. In analyzing what was most painful to him, it was the fact that the "secret" excluded him. My interpretation was that it forced him to feel like a "lone wolf", rejected by the pack. That disconnect was reflected on many levels psychically, including his dissociative, anxiety-riddled states as well as phobic reactions to various group situations. It was also a family trauma that was being perpetuated and enacted through Peter's exclusion from the group experience, almost as if he were being identified with the uncle in some way.

At this point in the analysis, making interpretations explicitly using group relations and socio- and systems-analytic concepts of tasks, role, boundary and authority helped Peter to understand his internal experience in terms of how it was impacted by his role within the family. This enabled him to more effectively assert his authority, as well as to relate to superiors and to maintain boundaries at work. Also, noting the connection to the collective trauma of hunger, though several generations earlier, as the original catalyst to patterns of emigration and family and individual upheaval has been useful in validating his sense of self and identity, and, therefore, supported integration and access to internal experience.

After first identifying the connection between the terror of external threats and internal wishes, fears and psychic processes, the analytic work can be aided by this framework in addressing the underlying internalized terror of one's own destructiveness to both self and others.

Jacob is by all standards a successful young adult with a bright future in his chosen profession. At the start of his treatment, he was stymied in his attempts to develop a lasting intimate relationship, something he greatly desired and valued, by his deeply rooted conflicts and ambivalence towards women. It was immediately evident that the frequent emotional unavailability of his mother, a child of a Holocaust survivor, played a crucial role in his expectations and behavior towards the women he dated. While his parents had what could be considered a successful marriage, despite their high levels of anxiety and frequent arguments, they both grew up in families that were less stable. Jacob's grandparents had experienced a great deal of loss and intergenerational trauma. Nevertheless, each successive generation experienced a degree of repair and sense of safety in its environment, so that Jacob and other family members of his generation were all poised to live productive and satisfying lives.

It was therefore quite puzzling and painful to Jacob that, despite his good looks, intelligence and well-developed social skills, he would make such bad choices in the women he dated, or generally avoid dating altogether. As treatment evolved, it became clear that Jacob's relationship with his older sister, whom he greatly admired and who in many ways served as an oedipal object—especially given his mother's emotional distance—had an important role in his psychic dilemma. As Jacob began puberty, his sister, a recent college graduate, developed ovarian cancer. While she responded well to the treatment and has since been able to resume her life, this was obviously a traumatic experience for her and the family, with continuing reverberations regarding her loss of fertility. The impact of this experience on Jacob has clearly many facets and derivatives, including his professional interests, heightened most likely by sharing a bedroom with his sister for a prolonged period as she was entering puberty.

Our work on the impact of these experiences, among others, enabled Jacob to become more aware of his tendency to feel overly guilty and to fear his underlying rage and aggression and its potential for destructiveness. Additionally, its relevance to issues and conflicts related to his sexuality became more evident. Jacob also tended to overreact to a range of situations in which he anticipated the most negative outcome possible as he paradoxically experienced greater success and was moving towards his longer-term goals. Despite feeling that his treatment was important and meaningful, as well as responsible for the significant progress in his personal life—he was happily living with a woman he intends to marry—he remained conflicted about deepening the work and moving into an analysis from a twice-weekly psychotherapy.

The identification of the masochistic, self-punitive component to Jacob's tendencies led us to the impact of a part of his family history. That is that his paternal grandmother was the product of a rape at a time and place in Europe, a generation before the Holocaust, when Jews were also subjected to a great deal of brutality. Exploring this piece of family history led to a better understanding of how Jacob experienced his male identity. Looking at how he was affected by intergenerational transmissions about masculinity opened the path to the deeper exploration that, up to that point, had not had signposts that resonated for him.

The clinician's sensitivity to the relationship between destructiveness emanating from external forces—which, unfortunately, too often has occurred through the aggression of one group of people towards another—and the process of internalization leading to the fear of one's own aggression and destructiveness is key to psychoanalytic work. Our openness to understanding the unconscious dynamics of groups and their interrelationship with the underlying forces within the psyches of our patients is therefore crucial to our effectiveness. Bion seems to have understood this in turning his attention to both individual and group unconscious processes related to trauma.

As psychoanalysts, as well as in our personal and professional lives as group members in a family, institute(s) and other organizations—as well as citizens in a society whose democratic values and principles are being challenged—we are continuing to struggle with the traumas of past and present. It therefore behooves us to continue to further develop tools that link the past to the present, as well as the individual to the group, in order to deepen and strengthen our understanding and effectiveness in all roles, arenas and levels impacting our current reality and experience.

References

Auerhahn, N.C. & Laub, D. (1998). The primal scene of atrocity: The dynamic interplay between knowledge and fantasy of the holocaust in children of survivors. *Psychoanalytic Psychology*, 15: 360–377.

Berger, S.S. (2014). Whose trauma is it anyway? Furthering our understanding of its intergenerational transmission. *Journal of Infant, Child, and Adolescent Psychotherapy*, 13: 169–181.

Bergmann, M.S. & Jucovy, M.E., eds. (1982). *Generations of the Holocaust*. New York: Basic Books.

Bion, W.R. (1961). *Experience in Groups*. New York: Basic Books.

Blum, H.P. (1986). The concept of the reconstruction of trauma. *The Reconstruction of Trauma: Its Significance in Clinical Work*, A. Rothstein (ed.). New York: International Universities Press, 7–27.

Blum, H.P. (1987). The role of identification in the resolution of trauma: The Anna Freud Memorial Lecture. *Psychoanalytic Quarterly*, 56: 609–627.

Charles, M. (2012). *Working with Trauma: Lessons from Bion and Lacan*. New York: Jason Aronson.

Faimberg, H. (1988). The telescoping of generations: Genealogy of certain identifications. *Contemporary Psychoanalysis*, 24: 99–117.

Fraiberg, S., Adelson, E., & Shapiro, V. (1975). Ghosts in the nursery: A psychoanalytic approach to the problems of impaired infant-mother relationships. *Journal of the American Academy of Child Psychiatry*, 14: 387–421.

Freud, A. (1936/1966). *The Ego and the Mechanisms of Defense: The Writings of Anna Freud, Vol. 2*. New York: International University Press.

Fromm, M.G. (2011). *Lost in Transmission: Studies of Trauma Across Generations*. London: Karnac.

Gainsler-Salomon, I. (2014). Inheriting stress, *New York Times*. March 7.

Green, Z.G. & Molenkamp, R.J. (2005). The BART system of group and organizational analysis: Boundary, authority, role and task. doi:10.13140/RG.2.1.2488.5929.

Kestenberg, J.S. (1980). Psychoanalyses of children of survivors from the holocaust: Case presentations and assessment. *Journal of the American Psychoanalytic Association*, 28: 775–804.

Kestenberg, J.S. (1993). What a psychoanalyst learned from the holocaust and genocide. *International Journal of Psychoanalysis*, 74: 1117–1129.

Laub, D. (1998). The empty circle: Children of survivors and the limits of reconstruction. *Journal of the American Psychoanalytic Association*, 46: 507–529.

Oliner, M.M. (1996). External reality: The elusive dimension of psychoanalysis. *Psychoanalytic Quarterly*, 65: 267–300.

Van der Kolk, B., McFarlane, A. & Weisaeth, L., eds. (1996). *Traumatic Stress: The Effects of Overwhelming Experience on Mind, Body, and Society*. New York: Guilford Press.

White, K.P. (2002), Surviving hating and being hated: Some personal thoughts about racism from a psychoanalytic perspective. *Contemporary Psychoanalysis*, 38: 401–422.

Zaiden, H., Leshem, M. & Gainsler-Salomon, I. (2013), Prereproductive stress to female rats alters corticotrophin releasing factor type 1 expression in ova and behavior and brain corticotrophin releasing factor type 1 expression in offspring. *Biological Psychiatry*, 74: 680–687.

Chapter 11

Trauma, destruction and PTSD

Vignettes of resiliency and transformative potential

Helen K. Gediman

Post-traumatic stress disorder (PTSD), which I am regarding in this chapter as more or less synonymous with adult-onset trauma, is a complex area of deep concern for psychoanalysis despite recent attempts to oversimplify it as a traumatically induced, but not necessarily analyzable, meaningful symptom constellation related to early conflict and other areas of inner life. This polarized view of the condition, embedded more in the context of external traumatization than inner symbolic meaning diagnostically, finds its parallel, therapeutically, in an overload of accounts, such as that by Gerger et al. (2014) of "evidenced-based" and behavioral treatment methods (see Schachter, 2014, personal communication regarding the paucity of psychoanalytic and other psychodynamic studies of PTSD). Carr's (2011) study of adult-onset trauma in combat veterans of the Iraq War is an attempt to correct for the deficit. He argues for a psychoanalytically based intersubjective treatment of the overwhelming affect, particularly of shame, that this particular population has suffered. I agree with Carr that these treatments can be researched and added effectively to evidence-based methods. Like Carr's work, most clinical and theoretical psychoanalytic studies of PTSD today are intersubjectively and relationally based, and focus on adult-onset trauma in which the present compelling and forceful traumatic effect overwhelms cognitive capacity to symbolize past early trauma and to analyze meaningful connections between the two. Major proponents of this position (Boulanger, 2005, Boulanger, 2012; Peskin, 2012) advocate a non-interpretive, non-symbolic but empathic, mirroring treatment whose therapeutic action consists only of "bearing witness" to and validating the patient's subjective experience of current traumatization in the here and now. As essential as this approach is to PTSD treatment, these authors seem to be promoting the false binary of bearing witness to vs. interpretation of the meaning of adult-onset trauma. In fact, meaning can be established and additional therapeutic work done that both bears witness to the unspeakable once the patient's cognitive capacity is no longer overwhelmed and the capacity to mentalize and to understand the meaningful relationship between early childhood and adult-onset trauma is restored.

Two important exceptions to the external vs. internal, or relational vs. intrapsychic, false binary stand out. The first is the Third Annual Conference of the Five New York Societies of the International Psychoanalytic Association, "September 11th: Psychoanalytic Reflections in the Second Year" (November 9–10, 2002). The second, a clinical conference entitled "Trauma, Destruction and Transformative Potential", jointly sponsored in 2014 by the Confederation of Independent Psychoanalytic Societies (CIPS) and the North American Psychoanalytic Confederation (NAPsaC), was also held in New York City, at Battery Park in commemoration of the new museum memorial to losses from the World Trade Center bombings. Both emphasized the important connections between massive external trauma and inner psychological processes, and both inspired the vignettes I am about to present. This work is a highly expanded version of a paper that was in press at *The Journal of Clinical Psychoanalysis* shortly before the time that it ceased publication in 2003.

Following the 9/11 terrorist attacks on The World Trade Center I had served on a psychoanalytic network, The New York Disaster Counseling Coalition, dedicated to treating 9/11 victims and first responders. My first two vignettes involve patients who were referred by this network. They had been inside or in the immediate vicinity of the towers when they were attacked, and survived by their own efforts. My third vignette involves a patient who was self-referred and had lost and had to leave her home because its proximity to the catastrophe rendered it no longer habitable. These three micro studies span a large enough range of PTSD symptoms and contexts to permit me to sort out some important relations between past and present trauma; to suggest who is most likely to develop the condition; and to identify factors that promote resiliency and the positive transformative potential of even the most egregious experiences.

The three patients I treated for post-traumatic stress disorder shortly after 9/11 presented with serious acute symptoms, which reactivated old trauma and other longstanding problems that predated the World Trade Center attacks. My work focused as much as it could on longstanding issues as well as the issues that initially brought them to seek help. None were in treatment with me or anyone else previously. They all believed they were suffering from PTSD, but also acknowledged they had other "issues", although symptom relief by means of psychological contextualization of these issues did not become a goal for all of them. All three were within a block of Ground Zero when the attacks occurred, and all three were convinced at the time that they were going to die, imagining no effective escape from the devastation they had witnessed.

Survival guilt and activation of overwhelming aggression was, and had been for a long time, a prominent feature in two of the cases. The early emergence of these concerns and the anxieties they exacerbated in what they expected to be a short-term treatment of PTSD appeared to prompt early unilateral termination.

In the third case, longstanding issues were integrated easily into the treatment, and the patient's acute response to external disaster potentiated a psychoanalytic focus on internal psychic events that lasted three years. PTSD symptoms as such were not as important to the third patient, who had lost her home, as relief from the psychic pain brought about by the complex meanings that the symptoms have in contexts that had predated the trauma. All three cases illustrate various ways that severe present trauma and subsequent PTSD reactivate past trauma and conflicts, and suggest ways of analyzing and contextualizing trauma in terms of past, present and future meanings that would facilitate therapeutic gains beyond symptom remission. Additionally, all three cases illustrate what Pyles in "Trauma and the Fate of Nations" (this volume) believes is inevitable for victims of suicide bombings: The after effects are uniquely painful and traumatic because such destructive terrorism involves understanding that real hatred motivated the killer to prefer his own demise to your survival.

Patient A

The crisis intervention counselor at a Wall Street financial institution referred a 24-year-old woman employee to me for treatment of PTSD. I saw Patient A once weekly for three months, after which she terminated unilaterally. During the 9/11 attacks, rescuers had evacuated her from her office near the World Trade Center, but she had been convinced that she would never come out of the devastation alive. She worked across the street from Ground Zero, felt her own building shaking, was in total darkness for some time and was witness to the overwhelmingly destructive immediate aftermath of the attacks, including people throwing themselves off buildings and landing near her office window. Someone told her there had been a terrorist attack; but because she was in a *dissociative state* during her evacuative escape, she really could not organize her thoughts at the time, and then again later in order to fully grasp what was actually happening. Both Anderson and Diamond (this volume) have noted the critical importance of dissociative states in traumatic experiences. Patient A reported classic responses to severe trauma: dissociation; repetitive nightmares; a conviction that a war would soon bring about the end of the world; and a fear that she would die early in the Armageddon-like struggle. Her world destruction fantasies (note the connection between fantasy and trauma in Busch (this volume) were not dissimilar from the events actually occurring in her surround. Bass (2002), in his discussion of an earlier presentation of some of my material (Gediman, 2002), noted that the victims of the terrorist attack were most likely to respond with PTSD symptoms when the present trauma closely recapitulated a past one. This case comes as close as any I know to Pyles' conviction of the uniquely traumatic effects of the terrorism of suicide bombers, referred to above.

Patient A's own destructive, including self-destructive, impulses were particularly stirred up by her conviction that because the terrorists were suicide terrorists, they would find no cause for mercy. It would certainly be very interesting to study differences in the capacity for resiliency among those threatened by suicide terrorists and those at the mercy of other forms of extreme destructiveness of self and other annihilation. This kind of evidence-based data could only buttress with good clinical support what we already know from possibly less systematic psychoanalytic studies: that world destruction fantasies such as hers often represent a projection of feelings and impulses from her inner world onto an outer world that shares many surface similarities with it.

At the time she came to see me, Patient A was terrified about having to return to her reconstructed original office situated in a building that had housed a morgue after the attacks. Although she was largely uninformed about psychoanalytic and other forms of psychodynamic psychotherapy, she understood, from numerous media reports that were circulating around 2001, that her major complaint, recurrent nightmares, was treatable by "talk therapy". She was most tormented post-traumatically by a recurrent dream in which she was married to and had two children with her current boyfriend, who, she emphasized, was "an American Christian". It was the middle of World War III, and there was a visible barrier dividing the safe from the dangerous zones, suggestive, at least metaphorically, of corresponding internal splits and dissociations. In her dream, her children—she in fact had none—were on the safe side of the barrier, where, paradoxically, to me at least, there was poverty, no food, water or shelter, and extreme danger of extinction. On the dangerous side, there was plentiful food and water and no poverty; but this side was presided over by a malevolent and frightening man, whom she labeled the "Antichrist" or devil. Her husband wanted her children to go over to the dangerous Antichrist side so that they could get food and water. Then the Antichrist villain seduced her two children across the boundary into the dangerous zone inhabited by Christians, where the children were killed. Then she was continuously running and there was no one around. This dream occurred almost nightly after 9/11 up to the time of our brief psychoanalytic therapy.

It was only after Patient A had reported this dream, about two-thirds of the way into her first session, that she tentatively offered the information that she was a Muslim, but did not say from which country. It was only in response to questioning that I learned she was from Afghanistan, and that she seemed uneasy about my knowing that. In our remaining 11 sessions, she apparently changed her mind and talked extensively about her life and current concerns. She had escaped with her parents from Afghanistan to the US in 1979, at age three, surviving the ongoing war with Russia. Her feelings about escaping that war and surviving successfully were most crucial to unraveling the meaning of her dream. She was undoubtedly intrigued by the idea that dreams had meaning and were not simply PTSD symptoms to be expelled via talking. She had been brought up as Islamic, but was an American citizen and attended a

Catholic university in New York, where she majored in religious studies, and claimed to be equally interested in Islam, Christianity and Judaism. In the course of her studies, she learned that the Antichrist who appeared so mercilessly in her dream is the devil and will at some point come into this world as a leader whom everyone will follow because they will think he is God. In retrospect, I can see the potential psychoanalytic value of analyzing this dream material with Anderson's idea of splitting in mind. That is, the extraordinary destructiveness of the external trauma resulted not just in dissociation—which was too disorganizing to allow her normally intact potential for organized thinking and regulation of affect—but in internal splitting, personified in her dream by who is on which side of good and evil. Anderson believes that once the primary dissociation as an initial response to overwhelming external trauma is addressed and mastered, the inner conflicts can begin to be worked on bit-by-bit as they relate to earlier trauma and repressed conflict. Although a similar idea was on my mind, I could not carry it through as treatment during the brief time she permitted me. Nonetheless, some of my psychological speculation follows.

Patient A's father had run a profitable business in Afghanistan and was able to escape with his family, his money and his health at the time of the 1979 war with Russia. We need to keep in mind that she had escaped and survived twice: as a Muslim survivor of the Russian–Afghan war and as an American survivor of the World Trade Center that was attacked by Muslim suicide bombers. She could not dispel her conflicting ideas about how she, as both Muslin and American, thrived when others had been killed. Because of her intimate involvement with a Christian man, she felt disobedient toward her faith and her father and feared the loss of her father's love. Father, but not mother, expected that she, unlike her sister, would most definitely marry a Muslim from Afghanistan. Until her involvement with her Christian boyfriend, she had been the "good girl", the favorite daughter of her father, who was heartbroken that she worked in a large financial institution instead of joining him in the family business as his major partner. She felt like a criminal many times over, not only for escaping twice, but mainly for betraying her father, who now in fact thought it more important than ever that she marry a Muslim. Analysis of the dream, brief as it was, revealed that her engagement to a non-Muslim man reactivated longstanding conflicts around moving away from incestuous attachments to her father, symbolized now in national, racial and religious terms. To add to this picture of conflict, trauma and her attempts at reparation, her boyfriend, around the time of 9/11, had developed a blood clot in his brain, and then a stroke. The patient, who was convinced he was on his death bed, accepted an engagement ring from him and agreed to marry him, but kept this information secret from her father.

During the brief period of time that I saw her, 12 sessions, Patient A's "PTSD" symptoms remitted and she seemed to be extremely motivated to understand the symbolic connections of her terrifying dream to both her conflicts and anxieties about split loyalties and to her multiply determined survivor guilt. She initially sought treatment because she was told that simply talking about the nightmare could make it, as a PTSD symptom, go away. However, as she got into the material, she developed an authentic sense of wonderment regarding the connection of the dream to important conflictual areas in her life. I suggested that she believed she, like the children in the dream, had crossed the line, simply by virtue of being my patient. That is, she was a Muslim being helped by, if not a Christian, surely a non-Muslim. She said she no longer wanted to see her Christian boyfriend but wanted to marry a Muslim to make her father happy and to receive his love once more. To uphold that tradition, she would not now marry for love because Muslim traditions maintain that love develops after marriage, never before. "I don't want to go any further. I want to marry within my own culture." She simply did not return one day and did not respond to phone calls from me.

I am assuming that Patient A's fleeing had to do not just with my belonging to another culture but with her inability to deal with the guilt generated by her survival, and by both conscious and unconscious conflicts between her wish to marry a Christian and still maintain her father's love. I have also wondered if her mother and I, who were basically accepting of her, represented the Antichrist, the false "God" who provided refuge, nourishment and life—none of which was able to counteract her terror of losing her father's love and respect when she became the "bad" girl. My neutrality and acceptance of her dilemmas might then have run counter to her strong, albeit unconscious, need to be punished for wishes she experienced as unacceptable oedipal transgressions. Who were now the friends, who the enemies? Another likely source of her need for punishment, possibly the most likely, was the inevitable aggression stimulated by violent and truly life-threatening trauma. Had the treatment been more than the unfortunately brief one it turned out to be—in which the patient attempted to heal her own splits in order to avoid the much more difficult work of analyzing the relation between violent external trauma and violent inner conflicts—we would have learned, undoubtedly, about the multiple meanings of that aggression. Perhaps that overwhelming affect was part of a compromise formation involving self-defense against a vicious enemy as well as a revengeful wish to punish her "persecutors". In sum, her inner and outer worlds might be considered as mirroring versions of one another when it came to issues of destruction and self-destruction, and particularly of literally identifying with a real aggressor. From a conflict and compromise perspective, aggression had been stimulated as self-defense as well as a vengeful need to punish. This was the first of two cases—Patient B described below was the second—whom I saw briefly, and for whom I believe that the prospect of relief from survivor guilt was unbearable; therefore they both left treatment as an enactment that precluded the potential for full, effective analysis.

Patient B

Three months after the 9/11 disaster, a 27-year-old man was referred to me by his investment banking firm counselor because his PTSD symptoms of massive anxiety and paralysis of everyday work and social functioning could no longer be treated on the job by personnel affiliated with his company, and called for more intensive psychotherapy. I saw Patient B twice a week for two months. At the time of the terrorist attack, he had been in his office that was just across the street from Ground Zero. When his boss ordered all employees to get away from downtown, the patient left his building and tried to reach his mother by cell phone but couldn't. He started walking toward the East Side, then looked back and saw the dark cloud and started running. "I thought it was the end of all of us." Smoke and debris overtook everybody, as it became blacker and darker. Somebody grabbed him; he grabbed others. Everyone saw that the World Trade Center had fallen, and were running for their lives. After running about a hundred blocks, Patient B was finally able to contact his mother, who told him that the State Department and the Pentagon had been destroyed. He told his mother, and then his girlfriend, that he was under attack and could not imagine making it out of the disaster zone. However, with the help of complete strangers, he made it to safety, but never felt safe. He was home with his mother by 1:30, but could not go back to work for two weeks after his office had reopened.

Initially complaining of PTSD symptoms, which were becoming worse by the day, Patient B could not stop looking repeatedly at the television images of the attack and collapsing buildings, and was convinced that he would never get over his PTSD symptoms and that he would die. He said he could not deal with these conditions because they were taking over his life. His presenting symptoms included trouble leaving his apartment for days on end, heightened anxiety, stress and difficulties in getting back to normal functioning on his job, as well as exacerbations of somatic symptoms of asthma, allergies and eczema. He initially presented these complaints in "checklist" fashion, with no introspection linking his symptoms to inner experiences, traumatic or otherwise. However, in the next weeks, he began to contextualize the symptoms by relating them to earlier, similar life events and seemed gratified by the connections he had made.

Although Patient B was initially inarticulate with me, as he had complained he had become at work, he soon enough moved quite spontaneously, and on his own, into recalling guilt about earlier losses of peers who had succumbed to illness and accidents. He was obsessed with the belief that they suffered their fate because he had abandoned them. His intense anxieties and fears related to old feelings had been plaguing him since his senior year in high school when a classmate-friend had been diagnosed with cancer and eventually died. He visited his hospitalized friend every day, and was contemptuous of his classmates who did not visit their buddy. He felt morally superior to all of them, and could not comprehend why his actions of friendly dedication and devotion were not appreciated. In time his ill friend's parents began to tire of Patient B, he thought, because he was trying to claim too much credit for keeping his friend alive with his visits. The friend survived through graduation and attended the ceremony. Patient B refused to attend as a protest that would assert his moral superiority over his classmates who never visited their sick friend, and believed his obvious absence would stand as a statement to publicize how negligent his friend's parents were because they did not give him credit for prolonging their son's life. Something similar had occurred in relationship to Patient B's younger brother, toward whom he showed exaggerated loyalty. His brother had developed a precancerous condition of the colon, and his colon was removed. Patient B then went off to college, believing he had abandoned his ailing brother. These memories of survival and guilt certainly seemed reactivated by his successful fleeing of the deadly World Trade Center site. One would have to wonder if his dependence on strangers to rescue him from Ground Zero triggered these memories of his own attempts to rescue friends at an earlier time.

In our brief (two-month) treatment, Patient B's PTSD symptoms disappeared, his somatic symptoms cleared up and he had set up a very satisfactory relationship with his live-in girlfriend. Troubles began, however, on the job. He became inarticulate and inhibited, yet certain that because he had been the outstanding person in his department, he would be promoted simply for having great potential and not for anything special he had been doing. When the promotion was not offered, he was bewildered. When I tried to help him explore his expectations and disappointments in relation to the apparent indifference his ill friend's parents had displayed toward his "specialness" he became quite distressed, referred to his survivor guilt, and imagined his guilt was keeping him from being more proactive at work so as to guarantee the promotion. One day he informed me he no longer needed treatment and was going to try something else instead. That something else turned out to be a determined effort to be more communicative with his girlfriend. Like Patient A, he clung to the belief in what he had heard from the well-intentioned Wall Street referral network. Therefore, simply "talking" to a friend was as effective as medication and psychotherapy in promoting PTSD symptom relief.

I began to wonder if the neutrality inherent in the psychoanalytic attitude toward survival guilt in some traumatized patients could produce a kind of negative therapeutic reaction. My two patients, A and B, were both convinced that they had done something terrible just by virtue of unacceptable wishes: in Patient A's case largely incestuous, in Patient B's largely oedipal aggressive—*both triggered by being alive in the midst of the death and incomprehensibly destructive catastrophe actually inflicted by real enemies who truly hated them as Americans.* This presently real constellation inevitably reactivated earlier similar trauma and conflict. The rather rapid disappearance, in both cases, of tormenting PTSD symptoms relieved the survival guilt temporarily. However, that very symptom remission disturbed certain other components of the compromise: e.g., the function of tormenting memory as punishment for aggression. Ergo, this very symptom relief blocked any further therapeutic progress. While Patient A punished herself with nightmares, Patient B punished himself with nightmarish memories to deal with guilt over aggressive wishes toward close friends he wished to rescue. His very symptoms had taken on a persecutory character in the service of self-punitive needs. At the same time, he expressed a life-long wish that parental figures indulge him with the love and care that they appeared to lavish mainly on others. Initially, these two patients' burgeoning capacity to understand the roots and to otherwise contextualize the meaning of their symptoms provided immense relief. The far too brief introduction to insightful reflection put them in touch with guilt related to longstanding conflicts involving incestuous and aggressive wishes. Although I could find common meaning in the childhood and adult traumas within interpersonal or relational as well as intrapsychic conflicts, as was the case for Boulanger's and Peskin's patients, they were not yet ready for interpretive work because the sense of being presently overwhelmed ruled out a therapeutically effective interpretation of the meanings that emerged. Their reflections on the inner past lives seemed to provide a powerful incentive for them to leave treatment before we could even begin to reach the phase of working through the relation of PTSD symptoms to both earlier trauma and to severe and persistent underlying conflicts. It was becoming clearer than ever to me that the triggering of earlier inner trauma by present massive external destructive trauma was a complex matter that requires extensive study from psychoanalytic and other psychodynamic points of view in our treatment of PTSD.

Patient C

A 30-year-old self-referred woman presented with multiple traumas that many would diagnose as PTSD. However, unlike Patients A and B, her encounter with external traumata potentiated an analytic process. I saw Patient C three times a week in a treatment that lasted four years. On 9/11 she, her husband and their infant daughter were at home across the street from the World Trade Center. They heard the crashes and explosions of the attack, and were in total darkness and ignorance with no electricity or water for 40 minutes. This terrified Patient C, particularly in retrospect, in a deferred revision of the initial memories once she knew and felt the full impact of these privations. The family congregated with neighbors, all believing that their home had been bombed and that they might die. Police arrived, and evacuated Patient C and her family to a suburb with just one possession: a diaper bag.

For Patient C, the traumatic events of 9/11 became conflated with the pain and suffering of a series of terrible traumatic events that preceded the attacks, as well as with significant times during earlier developmental crises. Her daughter was born two months before 9/11, which left Patient C with extensive genital lacerations and infections. When reparative surgery was attempted, medical negligence was responsible for some serious genital mutilation which might require radical surgical measures, yet still not leave the damage fully repairable. Sexual intercourse was then medically prohibited. Just before her daughter's birth, Patient C's financially successful husband had been laid off from his lucrative investment banking job. After 9/11 they were living in a rural area in New England for about three months, during which time Patient C's husband commuted weekly to Wall Street to work on deals that might restore his good fortune. In December, she discovered that he had been having a love affair during his weekly stays in New York, so she picked up and left with their infant daughter to stay with her mother in the distant state where she had grown up.

A month later, Patient C returned to New York with her daughter, primarily for her own continued medical care, and they moved into a building in my neighborhood. While her husband resided elsewhere in the city, she financed their rent, food and clothing with money from a bank account that she held jointly with him and with credit cards that had been issued in both of their names. At the time of our initial consultation, she had had very little contact with her husband and did not know his address, having only a phone number he gave her to contact him in case of an emergency with their daughter. Fortunately, Patient C was a competent and attuned mother (I had seen her several times with the baby before she found a reliable sitter) and had been carrying the parenting load single-handedly and well, without respite or much sleep. Unfortunately, the baby developed serious kidney and urinary symptoms, and had to undergo many painful medical-surgical procedures, which were traumatic for both mother and baby. During the course of the analytic treatment, the baby, like her mother, was never out of the woods, medically speaking. Patient C's husband appeared on the scene dutifully once or twice a week, but had become remote, emotionally removed and noncommittal regarding any future financial or other plans for involvement or disinvolvement with his new family. He seemed unable to act responsibly with regard to anything that had happened to them. Patient C, in her struggle with apparently ceaseless trauma, was in an excruciatingly painful state of limbo. I hesitate to designate her response as PTSD because it exemplifies another frequently found sequel to multiple traumas: an increased capacity of her ego to master intensely felt psychic pain. She was, in a word, resilient—the key, I believe, to optimal transformative potential for successful treatment responses following violent adult-onset external traumatization.

When Patient C began a thrice-weekly analytic treatment, she did very well. She suffered no survivor guilt, and chose to focus mainly on her husband's "change of character", as well as her denial of how he had been all along. It looked as though the marriage would either terminate or be sustained, mainly because both parents cared about their child's well-being. It did indeed end. Our work then focused on how current multiple traumata reactivated Patient C's serious early life disruptions, especially those related to her parents' marital breakup. At that time, Patient C and her brother, aged six and four, were sent to live with their loving but eccentric father so that their mother could be free to engage in love affairs. When she was 13, her mother made a new romantic connection, father left town and mother invited the children to live with her briefly, but then implemented a plan to settle Patient C and her younger brother in their own town house, a few miles from mother's new home. Patient C felt humiliated because everyone would think that she had been abandoned and banished from a normal family life. Mother rationalized that she could, with this incredible arrangement, conduct an unimpeded sexual life with her new paramour, and that Patient C could learn skills of independence and self-sufficiency. Patient C's mastery of this shocking situation might very well have laid the groundwork for her later competency as a mother. That is, as she relived, she also aimed to master the trauma of humiliation from abandonment and banishment in the interest of first her mother's, and then her own husband's sexual freedom. She of course connected her own genital damage and the medical threat to her daughter's well-being, which both occurred contiguously, to abandonments in which someone important left her to have better sex in their lives.

In the period following 9/11, Patient C, unlike Patients A and B, persevered and showed no sign of wanting to bolt treatment, perhaps because she suffered no conscious survivor guilt. Additionally, she is extremely bright, intellectually creative, psychologically minded, a free spirit and incredibly courageous. One predicts she might continue to develop and grow despite, or maybe even because of, such horrible multiple trauma that she is determined to master, just as she had to deal with a split family and an erratic mother and father earlier in life. Transference developed predictably; she did not flinch at hard work in her efforts to attain insight, support and means of mastery. She was able to understand the meanings of her present repetitions of past trauma in what analytic therapists aim for in helping their patients expand self-awareness.

I hope my three brief vignettes can teach us something about the relation of PTSD to earlier trauma. We could then understand a little more about how survivor guilt and the negative therapeutic reaction interfere with the treatment of currently instigated PTSD when the syndrome is treated without the benefit of in-depth analysis of the earlier traumatic and conflictual life experiences it inevitably reactivates. And I hope my limited material can shed light on the fact that objectively severe trauma can in some instances provide the conditions for a more favorable analysis than can traumas that are objectively less severe, albeit subjectively more severe, when they replicate certain aspects of survival guilt histories. Alan Bass has emphasized what I believe to be the distinguishing factor between negative and positive therapeutic outcomes with traumatized patients: the degree to which an overwhelming encounter with an external situation of unbounded inescapable destructiveness replicates the worst internal situation. The closer the replication, the worse the outcome: ergo, the limit of the benefits of treatment for Patients A and B, and the positive progression in the treatment of Patient C.

References

Bass, A. (2002). Discussion of Panel 3, Third Annual Conference of the Five New York Societies of the International Psychoanalytic Association, "September 11th: Psychoanalytic Reflections in the Second Year". New York City, November 10.

Boulanger, G. (2005). From voyeur to witness: recapturing symbolic functioning after massive psychic trauma. *Psychoanalytic Psychology*, 22: 21–31.

Boulanger, C. (2012). Plea for a measure of imagination: Commentary on paper by Harvey Peskin. *Psychoanalytic Dialogues*, 22: 206–210.

Carr, R.B. (2011). Combat and human existence: Toward an intersubjective approach to combat-related PTSD. *Psychoanalytic Psychology*, 28: 471–496.

Gediman, H.K. (2002). Trauma 9/11: PTSD and reactivation of earlier disturbance. Presented in a Panel at the Third Annual Conference of the Five New York Societies of the International Psychoanalytic Association, "September 11th: Psychoanalytic Reflections in the Second Year". New York City, November 10.

Gerger, H., Munder, T., Gemperli, A., Nuesch, F., Trelle, S., Juni, P. & Barth, J. (2014). Integrating fragmented evidence by network meta-analysis: Relative effectiveness of psychological interventions for adults with post-traumatic stress disorder. *Psychological Medicine*, 44: 3151–3164.

Peskin, H. (2012). "Man is a wolf to man": Disorders of dehumanization in psychoanalysis. *Psychoanalytic Dialogues*, 22: 190–205.

Shachter, J. (2014). Personal communication, May 18.

Chapter 12

Moral injury, the moral defense, and the collapse of emotional containment

An intersubjective alternative to PTSD in the treatment of wartime trauma

Thomas P. Helscher

No experience has challenged the limits of the psyche's capacity to register and make meaning out of our individual and collective experience like the destruction wrought by war. Primarily in its effects on combatants, but also on those connected to the veterans of war—parents, spouses, loved ones, children, the communities affected—war is responsible for massive, wide-spread and long-lasting trauma, and its catastrophic effects have necessitated diverse responses throughout history designed to mitigate and to heal these wounds of war. In a recent book, *The Theater of War* (2015), Bryan Doerries speculates that many of the most important Greek tragedies were written and performed by and for veterans of combat, and were designed to help a society process the psychological effects of the loss of loved ones, the guilt and shame of what one did and didn't do during battle, and the general horror of what humans were capable of inflicting on one another. In recent times, scholars, physicians, psychologists and psychoanalysts have studied and attempted to describe the consequences of training men (and occasionally women) to suspend our universal moral inhibition against killing and deliberately inflicting harm on others.

As David Morris outlines in *The Evil Hours: A Biography of Post-Traumatic Stress Disorder* (2015), perhaps our most important diagnostic category for identifying and treating trauma grew out of the struggle of Vietnam veterans to understand and get help for recurrent and devastating psychological symptoms that were either undiagnosed or misdiagnosed by the military's physicians, psychiatrists, psychologists and the Veterans' Administration responsible for treating them.

Most recently, there has been a movement away from simply focusing on the psychiatric symptoms covered by the diagnosis PTSD to an exploration of something called "moral injury". In an article entitled "Mad, Bad, Sad: What Has Really Happened to America's Soldiers?" (2012), Nan Levinson writes of moral injury:

> It's a concept in progress, defined as the result of taking part in or witnessing something of consequence that you find wrong, something which violates your deeply held beliefs about yourself and your role in the world. For a moment, at least, *you become what you never wanted to be.* While the symptoms and causes may overlap with PTSD, *moral injury arises from what you did or failed to do, rather than from what was done to you. It's a sickness of the heart more than the head.* (my italics)

At the heart of moral injury lies an intolerable identification with the internalized bad object, which, when coupled with the collapse of the good internal object, leaves the person in the grip of potentially suicidal despair. One of the most difficult therapeutic tasks for the morally injured individual is the need to reconcile his sense of himself as a good and decent person, and his sense that the world is a fundamentally good and fair place, with what he has been forced by his military service to do or to witness. In a recent collection of personal accounts by soldiers of such moral conflict, *The Things They Cannot Say: Stories Soldiers Won't Tell You About What They've Seen, Done or Failed to Do in War* (2013), Kevin Sites details the crippling guilt that constitutes one of the major factors in moral injury. Moral injury represents what Levinson describes here as a "sickness of the heart".

It is possible to have "moral injury" without suffering the full range of symptoms of PTSD. In a study designed to differentiate PTSD symptoms from moral injury, Litz et al. (2009, p. 697) found that "active potentially morally injurious roles had significantly smaller association with hyperarousal than being the target of the life threat" and that "combat guilt is largely associated for re-experiencing and avoidance symptoms, but not arousal symptoms". Other early surveys of moral injury, such as that by Dombo et al. in "The Trauma of Moral Injury: Beyond the Battlefield" (2013), also emphasize the moral, spiritual and psychological damage of combat instead of the merely psychiatric symptoms of PTSD.

PTSD occurs typically in response to prolonged or extreme trauma, and is a fear-victim reaction to danger. On the other hand, Jonathan Shay (2014), who was one of the earliest to address the plight of the Vietnam veterans and has become one of the most important advocates for this new diagnostic category, describes "moral injury" as an insidious secondary infection or toxicity that poisons a person's psychological or moral well-being, and argues that it is particularly prevalent among those who have served in combat. The concept of "moral injury" remains at this time an unofficial diagnosis for both the American Psychiatric Association (APA) in its *Diagnostic and Statistical Manual of Mental Disorders* (DSM 5) and the Department of Veteran Affairs; yet the latter has begun an extensive, long-term study to outline its prevalence among returning veterans.

What I would like to offer in this chapter is a description of this new clinical concept of moral injury, drawing in particular from the first object relations theorists, whose understanding of trauma grew directly out of their experience with the devastating effects of combat. I believe that by combining the work of the work of Klein, Fairbairn, Winnicott and Bion, we can create a way of understanding and addressing the psychic devastation wrought by war that constitutes moral injury. I think such a clinical understanding is critical for psychoanalysis at this moment of a paradigm shift that acknowledges the powerful effects of the relational field—whether defined as the familial environment of the infant; the social, cultural and political field of intuitions such as school and army; or the analytic field created by the intersection of the subjectivities of analyst and patient—for both pathological and therapeutic ends. Such an understanding seems the logical extension of the object relations thinking of Fairbairn, Winnicott, Klein and Bion.

In an article entitled "The Repression and the Return of Bad Objects (with Special Reference to the 'War Neuroses')"—written following his experiences supervising the treatment of and evaluating traumatized World War II veterans eligibility for disability and pension benefits—Fairbairn (1943) offers a description of the developmental underpinnings for the concept of moral injury. Fairbairn's argument follows from the assumption of profound infantile helplessness and dependency, and the infant's omnipotent defenses against this overwhelming helplessness. For Fairbairn, in order to manage caregivers upon which he is utterly dependent for his survival, the baby resorts to internalizing the caregiving object through identification and then subjecting it to repression, thereby banishing it from consciousness. The existential and external threat of one's survival being dependent upon an unreliable and "libidinally" bad (i.e. frustrating and pain-inducing) object is mitigated by this identification and internalization. The identification—the bad object is me—creates an illusion of omnipotent control: If I'm the bad object, then I can do something about the badness by modifying myself. As Fairbairn describes it, the unconditional badness of the pain of reality that one can't control is transformed into the conditional badness of morality: I'm bad because I do bad things; and if it's my agency that creates badness, then I can change that by doing good things instead. By this sleight of hand, the infant turns a situation of intolerable helplessness which could lead to profound and crippling despair—or, worse yet, organismic panic in the face of the threat of annihilation by forces vastly larger than oneself—into a seemingly manageable moral dilemma: I got myself into this, and I can somehow get myself out of it. Or, as Fairbairn puts in more eloquently,

> If it be asked how it comes about that conditional badness is to be preferred to unconditional badness, the cogency of the answer may best be appreciated if the answer is framed in religious terms; for such terms provide the best representation of the adult mind of the situation as it presents itself to the child. *Framed in such terms, the answer is that it is*

> *better to be a sinner in a world ruled by God than to live in a world ruled by the Devil.* (1943, pp. 66–67, my italics)

The critical point here is the gap between the reality situation—profound infantile dependency and helplessness—and the precocious intellectual defense against an awareness of this reality that could prove psychologically devastating. This developmental gap, first described by Freud as *Hilflosigkeit*, is at the heart of psychological defenses such as splitting and projective identification, denial and, what Fairbairn calls here, the "moral defense".

If the "moral defense" represents the infantile attempt to preserve an essential feeling of safety and goodness, then we could say that "moral injury" represents the collapse of the good internal object and a regression to the terrifying realm of what Melanie Klein (1946) calls the "paranoid-schizoid" position. What results is a profound sense of terror, existential despair and moral confusion. The individual's capacity to find meaning and purpose in his experience is severely compromised. What is crucial for this understanding of moral injury is that at its core is a fundamental environmental failure. This is one crucial distinction we can draw between moral injury and PTSD. Moral injury is always relational. Some basic sense of moral authority has collapsed or been breached, and as a result the foundational sense of "innocence protected" has been lost. Eric Brenman describes such a regressive threat in Kleinian terms in *Recovery of the Lost Good Object* (2006).

We can begin to think of moral injury as the result of a demand made upon us in states of helplessness and/or powerlessness that so compromise our sense of what is just, fair or good that it damages our basic sense of the world being a place that makes sense. To preserve the possibility of goodness—to protect the good object or the good mother in Fairbairn's terms, we take upon ourselves a moral judgment of "we are bad", which at its extreme (one might say psychotic) limit might involve a phantasy that the only way to protect and preserve the possibility of goodness is to do away with oneself. Obviously, Fairbairn's understanding of internalization of bad objects as a response to real environmental failures differs radically from Klein's understanding of splitting as a response to constitutional envy as a representative of the death instinct projected outward onto reality. In a similar vein, my reading of moral injury also differs significantly from more recent uses of the term that take a more classically Kleinian position concerning the role of the perpetrator and the guilt and shame that result from the awareness of having done "bad" things (Litz et al., 2009).

I worked with a suicidal borderline patient who, prior to coming to me, had made repeated serious attempts, and for a six-month period of the analysis made repeated serious threats to kill herself. Over time, we came to understand her suicidality as an attempt to preserve the good object by taking upon herself all the badness and doing away with it. As a result of a traumatic childhood and adolescence that involved living on the streets and turning tricks to support herself, she came to believe that the world was fundamentally corrupt—ruled by the devil in Fairbairn's terms. Everything you could do to survive represented some form of prostitution, and innocence and goodness could only be preserved by her sacrifice. After a six-year analysis, five times a week, this woman was no longer suicidal, had given up her antidepressants and was in a stable long-term relationship. Perhaps not surprisingly, following her analysis she went to divinity school to train for the ministry.

One could argue that the ambiguity at the heart of the term "moral injury"—who is injuring whom?—points to this problem of agency implied in Fairbairn's concept of the "moral defense". Certainly this is Jonathan Shay's conceptualization of "moral injury" (2014), since he believes it most often can be traced to the failure of the military leaders or civilian authorities—the institutional environment—that compels the individual soldier to act in ways that violate our basic sense of goodness. Although it's tempting to assert that simply requiring people to kill in itself constitutes a form of "moral injury", the situation is more complicated than that, as West Point professor of psychology and former US Army Ranger Dave Grossman argues in *On Killing: The Psychological Cost of Learning to Kill in War and Society* (1995).

Moral injury grows out of situations in which we are compelled, encouraged, expected to inflict violence or terror upon others, either intentionally or by accident: for example the killing of innocent civilians in situations of danger and uncertainty; or perhaps to passively witness and thereby render ourselves complicit in the killing of others. In *The Things They Cannot Say*, Kevin Sites begins with his personal account of what I would describe as his moral injury as the result of being a war correspondent:

> War's most cunning trick, it seemed, was the war it seeded within me. I wanted to cling to the concept of my own goodness, but the choices I had made during war seemed to indicate something else entirely: a man who was at best oblivious and at worst heartless. (2013, pp. 1–2)

Sites goes on to describe the events that led to this war within. On one occasion he videotapes a mortar shell exploding and wounding a producer he is working with at the time—the guilt growing out of his conflict between the demands of his profession, capturing "dramatic and rare footage, a seldom-captured incoming round and its casualty, the ultimate cause and effect" (2013, p. 4), and the demand of his conscience to drop everything and rush to the producer's aid. The dilemma is not eased by the producer's insistence, even as he bleeds, that the videographer capture his bleeding on film. In a second instance, in reference to a terminally wounded Iraqi man in his last agonizing minutes, he is asked by a soldier, "Are you going to videotape me if I shoot him?" (p. 6). Rather than risk the inquiry likely to be triggered by being videotaped, the soldier walks away and leaves the dying man in his suffering. Sites moves closer to the man and notices at close proximity that "the right side of his head is missing" (p. 6). In response to the question, he tells the marine:

> "Of course I am, that's my job," but as the words come out of my mouth, I'm wondering why I can't just let the Marine finish the job without videotaping it. Doubtless, the man is going to die. Why not let it be without more suffering? (2013, p. 7)

The dilemma Sites describes, and his response in the heat of the moment, represents the moral injury, and leads to the debilitating sense of guilt, depression and sleeplessness he describes returning from the war with, and result from the impossible demands of the situation that damage his capacity to make sense of his experience. It's important to observe that his symptoms, which he diagnoses as PTSD, result not from a particular threat to his life or personal safety, but from his moral conflict over what he did or witnessed, and thereby colluded in. This distinction is at the heart of moral injury as distinct from PTSD.

In this situation, the moral dilemma becomes more intense once the soldiers walk away, leaving Sites alone with the dying Iraqi man. We see the other face of moral injury: In addition to the impossible moral complexity of determining the "right" action at any given moment is the profound and debilitating sense of helplessness. This sense of helplessness, coupled with a profound sense of responsibility for the man's fate, deepens the journalist's sense of guilt:

> The two of them [Marines] walk on and leave me with alone with the Iraqi man with half a head missing. I look at him. He's still breathing, still bleeding. What's left of his life is in my hands now. I wonder if this is the worse way to die, alone with no one who can even understand your last words, if you have any. I wonder if I should've let the Marine shoot him. I don't know if he's suffering terribly or if that sniper's bullet removed any sense of pain or awareness along with that part of his head. *I wonder how I became the final arbiter of the last moments of his existence.* I look at him again and realize we are alone in this place together. The Marines are gone; there's no one else around. This Iraqi man, dressed in civilian clothes, most likely in his mid to late fifties, has no weapon by his side and perhaps he never did. He is almost certainly someone's father, maybe even a grandfather, but there's no one around him now, only me. He will die lying on the ground as a stranger holding a video camera looks over him. But I can't let that happen. It's just not right. So here is what I do instead: I walk away. (Sites, 2013, p. 7, my italics)

This moment can be seen as capturing the conditions that make for moral injury:

Profound helplessness in the face of extreme forces of manmade violence, mayhem, lethal destruction—"While he looked complete from a distance, a Marine sniper had fired a round through his eyeball, taking much of his skull and brain through the exit wound in the back" (Sites, 2013, p. 6). While such helplessness in the face of natural disasters may be traumatizing and induce PTSD, I would argue that only those situations created by human agency can result in moral injury, since it necessarily involves some confusion, conflict and/or shame and guilt about one's agency in a given situation.

1 The most extreme consequences imaginable: the experience of a man's last moments ("I wonder how I became the final arbiter of his last moments of his existence").
2 Tension between the demands of one's institutional role and one's moral sense of what is the right thing to do.

Finally, Sites describes a situation in which he films prisoners being executed in the field, and, by choosing to censor his videotaped evidence, unwittingly sets up another prisoner to be executed as the remaining witness.

> When I had bumbled out of the mosque with my videotape to seek justice for one summary execution, I had set the stage for another by ignoring the obvious probability that it would happen again. And it did. Had I simply walked Nidal out of the mosque, he might've lived. … To this day, I can't begin to fathom how I could have been so stupid … His death is the pinnacle in the case against me. (2013, p. 13)

To summarize then, we can think of the particular "moral injury" inflicted by war as the shattering of what Fairbairn describes as the necessary illusion of psychic health in early development—the world is ruled by God not the devil—a psychic devastation compounded by our necessary defense against overwhelming helplessness in the form of our identification with the bad object. We have become, in the words of Nan Levinson "what [we] never wanted to be"—a bad person doing the devil's business. Following "moral injury", both the world and the self become demonic in Fairbairn's sense: We lose the capacity to trust, to feel safe, to drink in the good object, which might help us to understand the extremely high suicide rates among returning combat veterans.

In "The Life and Lonely Death of Noah Pierce" in the Fall 2008 issue of *The Virginia Quarterly Review* (*VQR*), Ashley Gilbertson described the descent into madness and the suicide of a young man returning from Iraq.[1] His breakdown, while exacerbated by severe PTSD symptoms, seems better understood in terms of the breakdown of the moral order of the internal world characteristic of "moral injury".

> "It's kind of like the devil followed him home and wouldn't let him be," [his stepfather] Tom Softich told me.
>
> He was standing in ankle-deep water by Lake Vermilion, not far from the Canadian border, where he used to come with Noah to a tiny shack they'd built for hunting and fishing. "He was starting to say Satan had more power than God, right before he shot himself, but I told him that's not true, it's only if you let him. Noah was starting to think Satan was in control of everything, and I guess he is, if you let him."

Shortly before he kills himself, Pierce writes a poem trying to capture his state of mind:

> Two tours in Iraq,
> was it right?,
> was it wrong?,
> I don't know,
> My Anger,
> destined me to hell,
> now I drink,
> now I drink & cry,
> re-live my life when asleep,
> so many dead,
> so many killed,
> Now I question god,
> Is it dis-believe,
> or is it fear,
> I don't know,
> Don't want to die,
> Don't want to live,
> but should be dead,
> I'm already in hell,
> Two tours in Iraq.

Before committing suicide, Noah attacks his image—stabbing the face in his photo IDs, punching out the rear view mirror in his truck. And he leaves a suicide note:

> "Time's finally up," he wrote, "I am not a good person, I have done bad things. I have taken lives, now it's time to take mine."

Noah's breakdown manifests itself in this moment as a profound split between the "bad" Noah who deserves to be punished, his face shattered, and the "good" punishing Noah who serves an avenging angel—executing himself to preserve the possibility of goodness in the world. The logic of moral injury at its extreme limit—one's own agency turned against the self to extinguish itself. His execution by his own hand serves to protect for example the mother he lies to about going off to kill himself, or the sister he has attacked recently.

What I believe we see in cases of profound moral injury such as that suffered by Noah Pierce is a psychological devastation of the capacity to feel alive, to feel safe, to feel meaningful, to feel that the world is a place worth being in. It represents an injury to one's basic sense of being connected to others in a meaningful way. This rupture of the basic social contract helps us distinguish moral injury from PTSD, which represents instead an organismic and self-focused response to a profound threat to one's survival. Moral injury represents a loss in the capacity to trust, love, make a meaningful connection with the Other. Ultimately, moral injury sits uneasily on the line between individual pathology and communal responsibility. Understanding moral injury as the devastating collapse of a basic sense of trust and human connection helps us to understand the importance of the fraternal bond between soldiers in combat. This deep and powerful connection is the last loving link to a human and moral order, and therefore must be preserved at all costs. Freud describes this crucial fraternal bond in "Group Psychology and the Analysis of the Ego" (1921) as formed through identification between members of groups in the army as the social glue that holds groups together.

Another way of understanding the ambiguity of agency connected with moral injury is that it is a sign of the breakdown in the mind's capacity to use an internalized Other, what Bion describes as the container/contained relationship, to order experience—as subject and object become confused and the most fundamental epistemological categories blur together under the impact of overwhelming and unbearable levels of stimulation. Beyond the primitive splitting of self and Other into good and bad that is characteristic of the paranoid/schizoid position is an even more overwhelming and unbearable experience of the chaos of unrepresentable states of mind—terror, dread, fragmentation into bits. This overwhelming of the mind's capacity to symbolize adequately the experience of war is why moral injury is more than just PTSD: It doesn't have to be an experience that threatened one's survival and triggers the "fight or flight" neurological response of PTSD; it can also be triggered by something one has participated in or witnessed that exceeded one's mental categories—especially one's basic moral sense that the world is a relatively good and just place. The trauma of moral injury exceeds the capacity of the mind to process it effectively, and fundamental confusion is one result.

What I am arguing then is that at a more primitive, less object-related level, moral injury represents the collapse of mental and emotional containment altogether. As I suggested earlier, the moral defense represents a desperate attempt to preserve the categories of good and bad, and not just the good and bad object experiences themselves. Suicide in that context represents a final desperate attempt to stave off total chaos and irredeemable madness—to paraphrase Fairbairn, "better to die and preserve the phantasy of a world ruled by God (functioning as his appointed agent) than to live in a world ruled by the devil." To Fairbairn's notion of the moral defense as an omnipotent response to overwhelming infantile helplessness we should add then Bion's notion that the psychological catastrophe of war results from the collapse of mental and emotional containment, and the release of terrifying unmetabolized, proto-emotional mental states—what Bion calls "beta elements" (and what Fairbairn describes as the release of the repressed bad objects). Healing from wartime trauma and moral injury requires, therefore, a sympathetic mind that can contain projections of helplessness and terror, and that can metabolize and thereby detoxify traumatic experience. This reconstruction of what Bion describes as the container function is essential to sanity and to being able to reestablish love and trust. For Bion, what enables us to go on in the face of psychological catastrophe is psychological containment—and the consequences of its failure or breakdown is evacuation and collapse.

This kind of psychic catastrophe is perhaps illustrated in the moment Bion describes in "The Battle of Amiens" from his *War Memoirs* (1997), in which he witnesses his aide dying and calling out helplessly for his mother while Bion experiences the terror of not going on—collapsing and vomiting helplessly. In his article on Bion's development of the concept of thinking as psychological containment of unprocessed emotional experience, as Bion's response to his own need to process his war trauma, Lawrence Brown (2012) writes: "Pain is a sensory experience which awaits a name that will then permit the patient to 'suffer' it so that he may learn from experience" (p. 1211). Brown's point provides us one with important way of distinguishing dynamically or diagnostically between PTSD and moral injury: PTSD is a diagnosis of pains—not a meaningful experience to be suffered through until meaning can be made of it. PTSD is "a sensory experience which awaits a name that will permit the patient to 'suffer' it, so that he may learn from experience" (p. 1211). Suffering and learning from experience is the necessary process of dealing with the psychic devastation of moral injury. Although, as David Morris points out in *The Evil Hours,* his history of PTSD, the diagnostic category emerged out of Vietnam veterans' need to understand and make meaning out of their wartime trauma, particularly by sharing their experiences in groups with other veterans, the emphasis since then increasingly has been to focus on symptom removal rather than facilitate a therapeutic process that would allow one to "suffer them" so that the experience could be meaningfully integrated into one's life history. Morris describes in painful detail the re-traumatizing effect of such "manualized treatments" that discount the subjective experience of the veteran's attempt to create a meaningful narrative out of their suffering. Moral injury, on the other hand, is grounded in the premise that wartime trauma is deeply meaningful and profoundly relational, not merely physiological.

Thinking with the patient represents the mind's capacity to turn pain into productive and meaningful suffering: It represents Bion's revision of Freud's concept of dream work as designed to protect sleep into that capacity to transform raw emotional sensation—bodily pain—into meaningful experience. As Brown (2012) describes it:

> Bion's experiences also taught him about the importance of dreaming in the ability to distinguish between reality and phantasy. Endless bombardment and the deafening roar of battle resulted in sleep deprivation so that even though one might manage to sleep, "when you awoke you wondered whether you were dreaming" (Bion, 1997, p. 94). Thus, it was difficult to see how Freud's wish-fulfillment theory of dreams applied to combat situations "when the most appalling dreams … are much nicer than actual reality." In normal situations the "digestive" function of dreams allows the individual to metabolize experience by "dreaming" it, but when an overwhelming reality disables (Bion's version of) dream-work the "emotion-recording apparatus" of which Graves … spoke fails and reality becomes an interchangeable nightmare with phantasy. (p. 1197)

Following Bion, then, we might say that moral injury must involve some impairment of the capacity to dream—to emotionally process one's experience into meaningful narratives. Again, we can reflect upon the effect of moral injury as the disruption of the self's trajectory. If healthy psychic functioning depends upon the internalization of a productive couple—a child who feels and a mother who listens—then perhaps moral injury describes the damage done to the mind as emotional container, so that the world becomes a terrifying place filled with persecuting figures and aborted or stillborn attempts to make sense of one's emotional experience. Lacking the metabolizing capacity of a balanced mind, the morally injured individual is perpetually overwhelmed by both a flood of internal stimuli in the form of unprocessed traumatic memory—what Bion calls beta elements—and external stimuli in the form of sensory experiences that cannot be adequately fitted into a containing and endlessly dynamically fluctuating self-narrative.

Bion spent his lifetime processing his experience in World War I as a tank commander in multiple forms, with each iteration coming closer to representing the unrepresentable experience of being psychically disintegrated. As Carole Tarantelli notes in her article "'I Shall Be Blown to Bits': Towards Bion's Theory of Catastrophic Trauma" (2016), Bion's theories of catastrophic change are intimately linked to his attempts to make sense of his own wartime experiences. He first narrated his experiences immediately following the war in his diary *War Memoirs 1917–1919* (1997), a piece of writing he described as reparation for his not having written to his parents during the war. While it might be interesting to speculate what got in the way of the 19-year old Bion corresponding with his parents during this long and troubling experience in the military, it is clear that the diary is also Bion's very detailed, almost obsessional, attempt to capture his experience in the war. The focus, however, is not on his internal experience, although we get glimpses of his growing despair, his frustration with bad officers and bad food, his mental and physical exhaustion that increasingly sapped his courage and resolve. Instead we get detailed accounts of his company's movements around the Western Front, coupled with detailed, colored pencil drawings of the positions of the various forces, roads and villages. In a later pass at capturing his wartime trauma, Bion writes in his memoir *The Long Weekend: 1897–1919: Part of a Life* (1982), written near the end of his career and not published until eight years after his death, of the devastating effects of his wartime experience: "no protection [exists which is] more solid than a figment of the imagination" and that safety is a 'delusion'" (p. 147). Finally, in his last work, *A Memoir of the Future* (1991 [1975]), Bion shatters the form of the memoir into multiple voices to best represent his having been, as he describes it, "blown to bits." In that work, he notes that "nobody told me … that war service would change utterly my capacity to enjoy life" (p. 508). Like Noah Pierce, Bion suffers from the collapse of the good internal object to contain his experience and make it meaningful.

I think it would be helpful to look briefly at a clinical example of a recent veteran suffering the effects of moral injury, and in particular the damage it creates to one's capacity to make meaning of one's experience. This patient came to see me three years after being honorably discharged from the army, having served two tours of duty in Iraq, post-invasion. He was suffering from depression, but in particular from a sense of meaninglessness and a complete lack of direction for his life, despite having recently finished college and considering graduate work. Having grown up in a financially struggling large family, he had joined the army in order to get a scholarship to attend college at a time when the US was not at war. Three months after enlisting, the planes bring down the twin towers on September 11, 2001, and the country is plunged into war. He is rushed into infantry training to prepare for combat. Eighteen months later, having been trained as an infantryman, he finds himself in Falluja, Iraq, serving as a Military Policeman, enforcing curfew in a commandeered civilian vehicle. The institutional lines of authority, of training, of one's mission seem hopelessly fuzzy. They live in a neighborhood with young men across the street who fire at them from rooftops at night. One night after curfew, while riding with his commanding officer, they encounter a suspicious vehicle, which they order to pull over. Rather than pull over, the vehicle flees, and the commanding officer orders the soldier to try to shoot out the tires, as protocol dictates. When this fails, he orders the soldier to fire a warning shot through the rear window of the vehicle, again following the rules of engagement. The soldier does and the vehicle pulls over to the side of the road. The two soldiers approach and find that the passenger has been shot in the head and, while still alive, is holding pieces of his brain in his lap. From an apartment next to where the car has stopped, a crowd emerges—the dying man's distraught family it turns out. After much wailing, chaos and confusion, a story emerges. These were wedding singers returning from a wedding party, terrified that the unmarked civilian vehicle contained bandits, insurgents or hostile forces. The young soldier is devastated. The next day, he is forced to interview the family in the hospital when they come to collect the body to ensure there are no links between the dead man or his family and the insurgents. He can't move past this incident. Months later he is taken off the frontline for treatment for PTSD. After a brief and ineffective treatment, he is sent back to the front and to another tour of duty, where he witnesses the abuse of prisoners by untrained, drunken and occasionally sadistic soldiers. Again, he experiences recurrent severe symptoms of PTSD and is sent home for good. In his small hometown, he is welcomed as a hero, with a homecoming party, banners, public proclamations. And yet he feels like anything but a hero. He is given cognitive behavioral therapy (CBT) for his PTSD by a therapist who weeps and is visibly uncomfortable when he tells her of his wartime experiences. Haunted by guilt and a profound sense of betrayal and bitter disappointment with his military service, he seeks psychoanalytic therapy with the despairing sense that no one can or even should understand his experience. He is torn between an intellectual awareness that he was following orders when he killed the civilian and yet a profound sense of guilt that he will never be whole again. His is a portrait of moral injury. In a manic reparative attempt at restoring the lost good object, he becomes a radical animal rights advocate and strict vegetarian. He struggles to trust me in the transference as a good object—either I haven't been there and can't really understand, or I am complicit with the authorities who find ways of rationalizing what can't be made sense of. Part of him unconsciously wants to protect me from his toxic experience, by not sharing, by not forming an emotional connection with me. Like Noah Pierce, another part of him feels "I am not a good person, I have done bad things." He describes feeling like an exile in his home country, unable to feel he has a place where he belongs psychologically. He doesn't identify with his fellow veterans, but feels estranged from those like me who haven't been through his experience in Iraq. I feel both helpless and complicit—part of the society that has sent these young men to fight in our name.

If we think of moral injury as a trauma that disables our ability to make meaning of our experience, as raw pain that requires transformation into a meaningful and dynamic self-narrative, then we can see how psychoanalytic therapy represents the treatment most likely to effect meaningful change. Focusing on the psychiatric symptoms of PTSD risks leaving those suffering moral injury to wander like the Ancient Mariner in Samuel Taylor Coleridge's poem. In this story, the narrator has upset the moral order by wantonly killing a sea bird that annoyed him. This killing plunges the Ancient Mariner into a nightmare world, where he watches helplessly as his ship mates die of thirst, cursing him as they do. He is unable to sleep, tormented inside and out. The spell is broken only when he can come to see the beauty in the natural world that he had lost after his killing. He at first reviles the sea snakes on the water at night as "a thousand, thousand slimy things" that live on with him while his men die; like horrible bad part objects proliferating in the darkness; or, as what Bion calls, "bizarre objects". Later he is able to find the beauty in them: "Oh happy living things, no tongue/ their beauty might declare." Through his aesthetic appreciation of the sea snakes, he is filled with love again for the natural world, and is thus able to return home from his nightmare voyage. The Ancient Mariner returns to his home; yet instead of peace and forgetfulness, he finds himself compelled to tell his tale over and over:

> Since then, at an uncertain hour,
> That agony returns:
> And till my ghastly tale is told,
> This heart within me burns.
>
> I pass, like night, from land to land;
> I have strange power of speech;
> That moment that his face I see,
> I know the man that must hear me:
> To him my tale I teach.
> (Coleridge, 1834/1992)

The story the morally injured tells requires being received and transformed by the analyst serving as the representative of the society that sent him on his way. Through the repeated telling and the containment and transformation function provided by the analytic situation, the veteran can find his way home.

Note

1 Permission to quote from this article has been granted by the author. Please note that every effort has been made to contact the original publishers of the article. If anything is missing or incorrect in these quotations, please contact Routledge and we will endeavor to correct this in future printings.

References

Bion, W.R. (1982). *The Long Weekend: 1897–1919: Part of a Life*, F. Bion (ed.). London: Karnac.

Bion, W.R. (1991). *A Memoir of the Future*. 1975. London: Karnac.

Bion, W.R. (1997). *War Memoirs*. London: Karnac.

Brenman, E. (2006). *Recovery of the Lost Good Object*. London: Routledge.

Brown, L. (2012). Bion's discovery of alpha function: Thinking under fire on the battlefield and in the consulting room. *International Journal of Psychoanalysis*, 93: 1191–1214.

Coleridge, S.T. (1834/1992). The Rime of the Ancient Mariner. *The Rime of the Ancient Mariner and Other Poems*, S. Applebaum (ed.). Mineola, NY: Dover.

Doerries, B. (2015). *The Theater of War: What Ancient Greek Tragedies Can Teach us Today*. New York: Knopf.

Dombo, E., Gray, C. & Early, B. (2013). The trauma of moral injury: Beyond the battlefield. *Journal of Religion and Spirituality in Social Work: Social Thought*, 32 (3): 197–210.

Fairbairn, W.R.D. (1943). The repression and the return of bad objects (with special reference to the "war neuroses"). *Psychoanalytic Studies of the Personality*, D. Scharff & E. Birtles (eds.). London: Routledge.

Freud, S. (1921). Group psychology and the analysis of the ego. *Standard Edition 18*.

Gilbertson, A. (2008). The life and lonely death of Noah Pierce. *Virginia Quarterly Review* (Fall): 35–54.

Grossman, D. (1995). *On Killing: The Psychological Cost of Learning to Kill in War and Society*. New York: Little, Brown.

Klein, M. (1946). Notes on some schizoid mechanisms. *International Journal of Psychoanalysis*, 27: 99–111.

Levinson, N. (2012). Mad, bad, sad: What's really happened to America's soldiers? TomDispatch.com (June 28); http://www.tomdispatch.com/post/175563/tomgram%3A_nan_levinson%2C_moral_injury_and_american_war.

Litz, B., Stein, N., Delaney, E.Lebowitz, L., Nash, W., Silva, C. & Maguen, S. (2009). Moral injury and moral repair in war veterans: A preliminary model and intervention strategy. *Clinical Psychology Review*, 29: 695–706.

Morris, D. (2015). *The Evil Hours: A Biography of Post-Traumatic Stress Disorder*. Boston: Houghton Mifflin.

Shay, Jonathan (2014). Moral injury. *Psychoanalytic Psychology*, 31(2): 182–191.

Sites, K. (2013). *Things They Cannot Say: Stories Soldiers Won't Tell You about What They've Seen, Done or Failed to Do in War*. New York: HarperCollins.

Tarantelli, C. (2016). "I shall be blown to bits": Towards Bion's theory of catastrophic trauma. *The W.R. Bion Tradition*, H. Levine & G. Civitarese (eds.). London: Karnac.

Part IV

Technical issues/analytic resilience

Chapter 13

The clinical significance and problems of a traumaticentric view

Fred Busch

In this brief chapter on the destructive effects of trauma, and the transformative potential that psychoanalysis provides, I will focus on the issue of technique, and a troubling problem we've had.[1]

A brief history of the issues

For a long time in our history, psychoanalysts turned away from the destructive effects of traumatic early object relations. Freud's move from the seduction hypothesis to the theory of unconscious fantasies as the major cause of pathology sealed over the role of early object relations for some time. Within the United States, from the time of Spitz's (1945, 1946) work onward, studies showing the significant effect of early separations or parental neglect seemed to have a negligible effect on clinical thinking. Ambivalence followed by intolerance toward Kohut's early attempts to integrate intrapsychic conflicts (e.g., the vertical split) with the traumas of childhood seemed more the result of threat than reasoned thinking. It was a time when many American analysts, faced with the lasting imprint of significant events from infancy, childhood and adolescence, held on to the idea of conflict as the result of internal processes *only* in awkward ways through the 1980s (see Busch, 1999, pp. 19–50).

However, it is my impression that *as a necessary corrective to earlier notions we've gone overboard*, so that *a traumaticentric* view of pathology has taken over our field. Thus, I hear many analysts singularly emphasize empathic interpretations of trauma as the sole corrective in clinical work, without at some point addressing the fantasies, conflicts and defenses that inevitably develop in the face of trauma. I see this as a part of what Diamond (2017) described as an increasing "dyadic bias in psychoanalytic theory and technique" (p. 297). While I believe empathy with trauma is a necessary corrective in most analyses, as a singular approach it has the potential to lead patients into regressive states where they remain victims, overwhelmed by the reality of trauma, left alone with their coping fantasies that might seem shameful, frightening or just plain sick.

Thus, there is an increasing tendency to view our patients as primarily trauma victims rather than also victims of their own mind. We seem to view our primary goal as comfort rather than freedom from victimization (self and other) based upon a freer mind. We are losing contact with our more primitive side, and thus becoming less free to deal with these sides of our patients and the methods that might help them get there. In thinking about psychoanalysis, Green (1995) poignantly asks the question:

> What is its aim? Overcoming our primitive anxieties, to repair our objects damaged by our sinful evil? To ensure the need for security? To pursue the norms of adaptation? Or to be able to feel alive and to cathect the many possibilities offered by the diversity of life, despite its inevitable disappointments, sources of unhappiness and loads of pains? (p. 874)

Thus, while we've all come to understand the distorting interferences of trauma on development, I also believe that it is equally important to appreciate the individual meaning patients make of it. *A trauma isn't only an event*; it is also something that is processed within a complex network of ongoing fantasies and feelings, which include theories about the causation of the trauma and its solution, along with the intricate defenses against them. In short, it is the myriad ways our patients are driven to act out aspects of trauma, and the inner world built up around it, that need to be transformed via representations leading to increased mental structures and their holding capacity.

In the last 30 years, many in the United States believed it was through empathy alone that we could cure entrenched narcissistic character defenses resulting from childhood trauma. However, Anna Ornstein, in 2009, reflecting on the earlier work of self-psychologists, acknowledged:

> They have been confident that, in response to their empathic interpretive comments, the therapeutic process would deepen and a well-established self-object transference would make the use of these self-protective (defensive) structures unnecessary. However, accumulated clinical experience indicates that these well-established defensive psychological structures do not readily yield to change. (p. 468)

Two examples of working with traumatic disruptions within the analytic session

Example 1

A patient frantically calls the analyst a few minutes before her appointment, saying that there is a power failure and no trains are running. As she is speaking to him, the power is restored, and she abruptly ends the phone call.

The analyst takes a nap while waiting for the patient, who shows up halfway through the scheduled session in an agitated state. She curses the transit system, describes the haughty behavior of a ticket collector and eventually runs out of steam, ending by insisting the analyst is angry with her. It turns out this feeling, "the analyst would be angry", occurred immediately after she abruptly hung up on him when the power was restored. As the patient demands that her analyst come clean about his feelings, he starts to feel *irritated.* Musing about his nap, he is aware of feeling quite relaxed and alert in listening to her. Yet the patient is positive that she hurt the analyst's feelings when she abruptly stopped the phone call. She confesses that *it is the type of thing that would make her really angry.*

Rather than either (1) appreciating the patient's ability to recognize her own her projection, or (2) reflecting on his countertransference reaction of anger and its role in the patient's view of him, the analyst responds by questioning the patient's perceptions of him—i.e., YOU THINK YOUR VIEW IS TRUE BUT I KNOW WHAT'S TRUE. He tells the patient that he was calm, and in fact fell asleep while waiting for her. However, earlier the analyst had mused on the possibility that his sleeping was a withdrawal from the potential onslaught of anger he expected when his patient came in. The patient then comments, more calmly now, that she has noticed a change in his level of activity in the session. So, one might wonder if the analyst's denial of the patient's perception put the kibosh on her feeling that she may have picked up on some anger in the analyst's initial reaction. It is not clear how the ensuing material unfolds; but what emerges is that the patient feels that her analyst has been energetically with her in the past few days, and she views his decreased activity as a sign of his anger in response to her cutting him off on the phone.

The analyst understands the patient's reaction as based on the loss of his calming function when he was less vigorously responsive, which often led to her perception that he was being punitive. In thinking about this the analyst says he has *in mind a model scene, where the distress of a child, possibly after an agitating experience such as an unexpected separation, is attempting to establish a lively intimacy with a disinterested or aversive, possibly depressed, adult. Her efforts go unnoticed, and depletion threatens her fragile sense of self.*

The analyst continues:

> In a situation like this, where the weekend loomed and the transportation system had let her down so cruelly, she was in need of a welcome that included a degree of attunement to her state of agitation to be able to maintain her sense of connection to me. (Lichtenberg & Kindler, 1994, p. 416)

What I want to highlight is that by primarily viewing the patient's upset state as a repetition of a trauma, the patient's perception of the analyst's anger is negated, and her need to project her anger is left unappreciated. She is left as the victim of the bad analyst and bad parents, and her fear of something bad happening if she becomes aware of her anger, or the analyst's. Her attempt to see her own role in how she views the world is negated. Her use of her own mind is negated by the analyst's seemingly benign empathy. She is left without any sense of agency, like the cut-off power that makes her frantic. She remains dependent on the analyst's power to feel enlivened, while the power of her own thoughts is negated.

Example 2

I will now present a clinical vignette where a brief empathic breakdown because of a countertransference enactment on my part led to a rupture in the session. I hope to show how I see psychoanalysis *transforming* the destructive effects of trauma into meaningful growth of structure. I've come to the conclusion that meaningful growth in psychoanalysis comes from transforming what has been under-represented, or represented in simple and driven form, into complex representations that create the possibility of greater freedom of thought and feelings, along with the potential of greater self-awareness and self-reflection. Marilia Aisenstein has expressed this perspective will when she wrote:

> Analysis is uncompromising in relation to other therapies because it alone aims, other than bringing relief from a symptom, at aiding our patients to become, *or to become again, the principal agents in their own history and thought. Am I too bold in insisting that this is the sole inalienable freedom a human being possesses?* (2007, p. 1460, emphasis added)

My patient, Harold, was in his mid-forties, the director of a prestigious post-doctoral fellowship program in the biological sciences, and in his fourth year of analysis. He came into analysis because of anxiety and depression, and the beginning years of the analysis were characterized by Harold speaking in muted tones, with constant self-criticism.

Harold began this session enthusiastically talking about a great applicant for the fellowship. He was impressed with her application, and described his impression of her when he interviewed her as a perfect "10". In contrast to his usual restrained approach with applicants, he told her he would really like her to come to the fellowship. She was pleased by the offer, but noncommittal in that for personal reasons she was looking at fellowships in Berkeley. About a week later he wrote an e-mail telling her again that he'd like her to come, and that they had so much to offer her. He then said to me:

> It's something I've not done before, preferring to have the program sell itself. She wrote back, saying how flattered she was and how appreciative of the note. I was going to leave it at that, but then decided "what the

hell?" I wrote her back and said, "Why don't you just come to Boston—it's great here." It was so unlike my usual stance, but it was fun.

I found myself enjoying Harold's freedom to feel playful, spontaneous, and able to enjoy the sexual undertones of the interaction without withdrawing. This had been a major problem for him in the past. So, I said:

FB: It's like a seduction.

(I thought I would say this in the same playful way Harold was speaking. However, in retrospect, what I said might have sounded more authoritative. It was as if I was showing him something new, rather than enjoying what he figured out. However, I did not grasp this at the time. Even more striking was that I said anything; according to my usual technical stance, there was no reason to speak, since I could see that Harold had a newfound freedom to feel, act and observe all this.)

There was a brief pause before Harold started talking again, and when he did, it was as if all the life had been drained out of his voice. His animated account of his interaction with the applicant was replaced by hesitation and a deadened voice. After he spoke this way for some time I said:

FB: After I made my comment about it being like a seduction, I'm hearing a significant change in the liveliness of your voice.

This is a simple clarification. I generally find that it is important to first clarify what is going on, to see if the patient can also see it. If he can't there are various alternatives, but interpretation of the observation is not one of them. At times, a clarification itself can open up the patient's mind. Notice also my clarification is unsaturated, in that I'm only saying something went on after my remark.

HAROLD: I also noticed it, but for some reason couldn't say it. *(Now more animated.)* I was talking with Esther yesterday. *(Esther is a postdoctoral fellow in whom he is consistently disappointed; he has given her many projects that he feels are exciting, but she barely does them. He feels she does not appreciate how much he has given her.)* I laid out a plan for her for the next few years, and all she did was complain about how much work she has. Then during my discussion with Esther, Sam *(another postdoctoral fellow)* came in, and commented on the research design. I said to him, in a not very nice way, "Sam, that's obvious." I guess it's another example of how I stay distant from people.

(He then starts to describe various ways he feels he distances himself from others and from me. His readiness to take on blame in the face of irritation has been a familiar defense.)

FB: When I point out the change in your voice after my remark, your thoughts go to someone unappreciative of how much you offer, and how irritated you felt with someone who pointed out the obvious. *(The clarification.) I wonder* if it seems these feelings are related to my comment, but something seemed unsettling about them, which led to your inhibiting yourself and then blaming yourself for your distance, rather than blaming me.

(While Harold was talking, I found myself thinking of the experiences he talked about where, when he took pride in his burgeoning phallic narcissism, his mother would put him down.) One story seemed typical of his experience. Around age five, while playing in his back-yard, he saw a bird lying awkwardly in the grass. In his memory, he tended to the bird, and it eventually could fly away. He came running to his mother to tell her of the miraculous good deed he felt he had just performed, and his mother's response was to tell him to go wash his hands immediately, as the bird probably had some disease.

I also thought of his mother's rages, which led him to isolate himself from the family. At this point, as in the previous case, I could have made an empathic interpretation suggesting that my remark, like so many his mother made, didn't appreciate his ability to feel comfortable putting it all out there with this woman, and shutting down his feelings was like what he had to do so many times to avoid his mother's hostility and protect her fragility.

I was also musing on what was set off within me that led to my remark in the first place. What first came to mind was a letter I had just received from an editor of a journal who overrode her reviewers to summarily reject an article I submitted. In my remark to Harold I was the now the one who summarily dismissed his discovery.

However, I felt if I only empathized with how I put him down it would be the end of the story. He likely would have accepted it, but now I would be center stage, the one who knew everything that was going on in his mind. Therefore, it seemed important to help Harold gain mastery of the story, by primarily clarifying that the story ended after I spoke, and yet he blamed himself for it.

HAROLD: What you said was fine. You were just describing what I was talking about. Hmm! Maybe I just said that you said the obvious. But I didn't feel it. Yet, Sheila *(a co-worker)* has a habit of summing up what I say, and I know I hate it when she does that. So, I guess what you said was really to the point. I realize I'm afraid that if I say something critical to you, then you won't say anything again. I don't know why I'm thinking this, but I'm worried about not finding Jodie *(his wife)* attractive. When I saw her this morning, she looked so tired and washed out. But she really looked good once she got dressed and put on her makeup. Did I really have to say that? I guess I did. *(Brief pause.)* I realize there's been something in the back of my mind while I was just talking. It finally came to me. I was taking this English class as an undergraduate and we were reading one of the American classics *(which he mentioned)*. We were supposed to write a paper on this one novel, and I went to the professor and told him about my idea. *(The idea had to do with a character's seeing something and never wanting to go back to the way things had been.)* The professor's eyes lit up, like I had literally opened his eyes to something he hadn't seen before. He then spent the first five minutes of the class talking about how you could never tell from whom you might learn something. You know, I wasn't ever able to admit this at the time, but I felt disappointed that he wasn't able to say it was me. He made it seem like *he* saw something, rather than that it was me who saw it.

FB: Like me.

HAROLD: Yes, like you.

FB: I wonder if when you felt disappointed and angered with my comment, you worried that pointing out this unattractive side of me could drive me away.

HAROLD: *(After a pause.)* You mean like I felt toward my mother. Or do *I* mean like I felt toward my mother? I feel myself starting to withdraw again. I was really moved by what you said. I felt we're real partners here. I also felt some irritation with you. Then I felt, "Okay, enough for today." *(At this point, our time was up.)*

In this vignette, we see how my countertransference enactment leads to a rupture in the treatment alliance—a mini-trauma. Harold is aware of negative feelings toward me, but is *fearful of putting them into words.* My representing the affective change in Harold's voice after my remark—i.e., that is acknowledging *something* happened rather than saying what happened—leads Harold to freely associate to other interactions where he felt irritated with the way someone was reacting to him. Representing Harold's fear of telling me about these feelings when I made my remark leads to further associations as to why this might be. In my view, transformations in psychoanalysis can be seen in the greater freedom to represent thoughts and feelings that were unthinkable, unsaid and not felt. Harold's analytic progress can be seen in his changing what was enacted into thoughts and feelings that could be reflected upon. It took his analyst a bit longer to do the same.

Final thoughts

There are many methods we use that are a necessary part of any analysis. However, I think most analysts in the international community would agree with Elias and Elizabeth de Rochas Barros (2011) when they convey the idea that constructing representations is centrally important to contemporary psychoanalysis because representations are essential for thinking and storing emotional experience. Without representations, we are fated to reenact, while with representation we can play with ideas, flip them upside down or backwards—and in this way contemplate many possibilities. We are finding new ways to make representations meaningful to our patients, and more sophisticated explanations for why representations are important. Further, as Green (1975) pointed out, by building representations we "bind the inchoate" (p. 9), thus giving a container to the patient's content and "content to his container" (p. 7). While empathy for the patient's plight and acknowledgment of the role we may sometimes play in it are necessary parts of an analysis, what I've tried to point out today is that it is most often the beginning of the patient's story, not necessarily the end.

Note

1 An earlier version of this chapter was presented at the CIPS/NAPsaC Clinical Conference on Trauma, Destruction and Transformative Potential in New York City, May 2014.

References

Aisenstein, M. (2007). On therapeutic action. *Psychoanalytic Quarterly*, 76S: 1443–1461.

Busch, F. (1999). *Rethinking Clinical Technique*. Northvale, NJ: Aronson.

da Rocha Barros, E.M. & da Rocha Barros, E.L. (2011). Reflections on the clinical implications of symbolism. *International Journal of Psychoanalysis*, 92: 879–901.

Diamond, M. (2017). Recovering the father in mind and flesh. *Psychoanalytic Quarterly*, 86: 297–334.

Green, A. (1975). The analyst, symbolization and absence in the analytic setting (on changes in analytic practice and analytic experience): In memory of D.W. Winnicott. *International Journal of Psychoanalysis*, 56: 1–22.

Green, A. (1995). Has sexuality anything to do with psychoanalysis? *International Journal of Psychoanalysis*, 76: 871–883.

Lichtenberg, J.D. & Kindler, A.R. (1994). A motivational systems approach to the clinical experience. *Journal of the American Psychoanalytic Association*, 42: 405–420.

Ornstein, A. (2009). Do words still matter? Further comments on the interpretive process and the theory of change. *International Journal of Psychoanalytic Self Psychology*, 4(4): 466–484.

Spitz, R.A. (1945). Hospitalism: An inquiry into the genesis of psychiatric conditions in early childhood. *Psychoanalytic Study of the Child*, 1: 53–74.

Spitz, R.A. (1946). Hospitalism: A follow-up report on investigation described in volume 1, 1945. *Psychoanalytic Study of the Child*, 2: 113–117.

Chapter 14

Sources of internal psychic trauma

Maxine K. Anderson

I would like to focus my thoughts on sources of *inner* psychic trauma, how the mind may dismantle its own capacities to think and to feel human.[1]

A while ago a small group of colleagues was reading a paper which focused on the traumatic alienation and dehumanizing experience that many suffered in Nazi-occupied countries during the 1930–1945 era. Specifically, the paper dealt with how exclusions and degradations, such as from the rights and privileges of citizenship in one's country and local community, could trigger a parallel alienation within the self such that the individual feels lost and frozen in a dehumanized inner world. In reading this paper, we each had initially found it a difficult one to follow, getting lost at times, wondering what the point was. And as we came together to compare notes for the first 20–30 minutes of our meeting, each of us easily fell into a kind of despair, not so much focused on the paper it seemed but more on the current state of the physical world: That, for instance, we humans have finally done it, exploiting the biosphere, tipping the environment beyond salvation. We were each expressing a sense of inevitable doom. And as we spoke we confirmed and deepened this state of mind in each other. Finally we were able to realize that we had become completely identified with the state of mind being described in the paper, the bit-by-bit dismantling of the mind and the human spirit from thoughtful beings with fertile minds into paralyzed cogs caught in a frozen wasteland of despair, a wasteland that we had helped to create through collective neglect and indifference.

This realization that we had so identified with the effects of trauma so vividly described allowed us to regain distance from the bleakness, so that we could reflect upon having been caught in it rather than just being encased and paralyzed. While one of us spoke to this possibility, another recalled a recent documentary depicting a significant movement afoot amidst the community of North Korean defectors dedicated to communicating back to their families and communities about physical and mental life in the outside world (Frontline, 2014). What was being made clear was that once the outside view can be accessed and taken seriously an awakening of the mind becomes possible, and the propaganda about local life as a paradise, now so prolific in North Korea, can be seen to be a lie. The awakened mind can see that the starvation is real, that the well-stocked department stores in which nothing is for sale can be seen as cruel props to keep one numbed against the reality of an impoverishing, enslaving dictatorship. Once there is an awakening the self can make space for vitalizing passions and curiosity, and it can both perceive and become aroused against the lie.

As our study group began then to be able to view itself from outside the morass, we could see that we had fallen into a frozen envelope and had become temporarily overwhelmed by it. I bring this vignette as an illustration of the effects of trauma: *The numbing of the sensibilities to the degree that intuitive and reflective thought is lost and one becomes frozen in the flattened, dehumanized experience of "how it is and will be forever".*

The crucial aspect of this traumatic dismantling seems to be the collapse of the capacity for this wider humanizing view, a capacity that has been thought about from several perspectives. One view is that of reverie (Bion, 1963), that sturdy capacity to receive but not be overwhelmed by pain or distress. The sturdiness here is vital for the transformation of traumatic impact because it provides the capacity to see that traumatized/traumatizing state from afar, and thus to think about it rather than to remain immobilized by it. Other conceptual frameworks (Green, 1999; Hegel, 2003; Bass, 2000) suggest the crucial role of negation and 'otherness' in establishing that separate rescuing function: In its effort to remain quiescent the primordial self naturally opposes any disturbance, and thus attempts to evacuate or to negate the disturbance as "not me" into an "other" which then becomes the location and the perceived "source" of the disowned disturbance. Reverie and negation serve as attempts to maintain space for thought and differentiating growth.

Still, to the fragile self, seeking quiescence through the difference or separateness of the other is just as disturbing. We can sense this most vividly in our narcissistically encumbered patients, who feel so disturbed by anything new that they can neither learn nor grow. They frequently need to hold onto a sense of possessing the truth and to be in control of reality in order to counteract the terror of not being in control at all. And we frequently realize that in order to help these patients we must hold our sturdy separate view rather than comply with their demands for perfect alignment. Our wishes to be empathic and well-attuned are put to the test in these situations because our separate minded efforts may be felt only as our being mean, rigid and controlling in not offering soothing affirmation. As Bass suggests, it is essential that we be able to speak to this pain, but also hold the space for difference.

Several years ago I wrote about this experience in some detail (Anderson, 1999). In brief summary, a patient requesting changes in the analytic frame, presenting them as reasonable requests, dreamed repeatedly of a mad old woman very shortly after I complied with each of those requests. Our mutual efforts to understand those dream figures revealed that each of them was me the analyst "gone mad" for complying with the "request". That realization relieved my patient, who felt there was something very deep which needed to be addressed. And it suggested to both of us that I needed to refrain from compliance with those requests in order to engage in that deeper investigation. So a few weeks later when the same request for my compliance was made I refrained rather than complied, expecting she would also likely remember our mutual learning. But to my surprise all memory of that learning had entirely vanished for my patient; instead she became locked into a conviction, which felt increasingly to me as a penetrating accusation of my rigidity and cruelty in my non-compliance. We were in different mental worlds.

I felt left alone with the awareness derived from the learning from the dreams, of the need to be sturdy, not to become the "mad old woman" of the dreams in the face of the steady barrage of complaints. But in a way I was becoming mad, as her painful complaints about my non-compliance increasingly felt to me as eroding my trust in the learning from the dreams, such that I was coming to feel that her penetrating complaints were indeed declaring the truth about me. At one point, when we both seemed to be exhausted by this process, I asked my patient if the seemingly endless experience of her intensely held complaints about me was feeling too much for her to bear. To my surprise she immediately said "Don't give up on me," which I took, and she later affirmed, was her need that I remain sturdy in this endeavor, to keep the reverie and inquiry alive. With our continued work on helping her gain clarity about the pain of difference between our views, my patient was slowly able to emerge from her conviction and to become grateful as well for the earnest hard work we were both engaged in.

We were later able to see that she had felt enslaved by a cruel inner voice of doubt and condemnation about ever being able to grow or to change. Studying that experience of confrontation with this accusing inner voice led to several findings, one being that there are intensely opposing internal realities or psychic truths. The "either/or" mental world based on "difference as the enemy" fights mightily against the recognition of the quieter mental world based on embracing difference toward growth and change. Indeed, the complaints seemed to be wearying attacks upon my capacity to operate at the level of the quiet deeper truth as if trying to keep any appreciation of difference at bay. The deeper truth, as signaled by the lessons from the dreams, was gained only by enduring the accusations, which emanated from the unabated hatred of her internal disturbance. That endurance is vulnerable to our empathic wishes not to cause our patients pain, and in my experience we may not always be able to bear the cries and accusations to get to this deeper truth. Our wish to not cause pain may foreclose those efforts to endure to the depths.

Helped by my patient's comment of "Don't give up on me," both of us endured, and thus were able to recognize the underlying threat or trap for the thinking mind. This remained hidden behind the complaint. It could be thought of as a kind of terrorist threat: "Comply with my demand as if it were a reasonable request or, through my penetrating accusations, I will wither your sturdiness and thus invade and destroy your separately thinking mind." Even more succinctly, and perhaps darkly, we came to see it as: "Comply with my propaganda (that my hatred of disturbance is the only viable truth), or I will invade and destroy your capacity to see any other truth at all." Being able to hold this external view of the erosive complaint as a hidden threat against seeing wider truths aided me in helping my patient to escape from the grip of her own enslaving resistance against growth and change, her own North Korea. Those learnings have continued to help me with such entrenchments in subsequent years.

The hatred of difference, the insistence on a seamless, undisturbed reality may encumber us all. These very basic human tendencies, when entrenched and stifling, become imprisoning to growth, and indeed to our whole-mindedness. Our study group was debilitated by the reading, which we came to understand as our being overwhelmed by the mind-stripping trauma described so vividly in the paper. But we were also feeling swamped by the guilt of our own participation in the indifferent abuse and destruction of the physical environment. This guilt might also have related to the unconscious awareness of our complicity in the abuse of our own psychic environment, that is, our own hatred of disturbing difference. As adult professionals this could be exemplified in our stalwart refusals to seriously consider ideas or positions that challenge our deeply held theories or beliefs. Much of the time we can welcome new ideas with interest and curiosity. But at times, when we feel defensive or threatened or otherwise more loyal to the known rather than to the unknown, we may resort to the violence of the splitting processes, creating an "us" and "them" world in order to rid ourselves of these threatening differences. And when we resort to this internal violence we are being at best indifferent to the fragility of our fertile minds, so needed for learning and growth and openness to the new idea. So our narcissistic tendencies which make use of splitting and projection may traumatize our whole-minded functioning, making us both the perpetrators and the victims of our own internally generated trauma. This is part of the human paradox, and one worth holding in mind in a culture which values grasping and possession as strength rather than valuing evolution and uncertainty as wisdom.

Note

1 Portions of this chapter were originally presented at the CIPS/NAPsaC Clinical Conference on Trauma, Destruction and Transformative Potential in New York City, May, 2014.

References

Anderson, M. (1999). The pressure for enactment and the hatred of reality. *Journal of the American Psychoanalytic Association*, 47: 503–518.

Bass, A. (2000). *Difference and Disavowal: The Trauma of Eros*. Stanford, CA: Stanford University Press.

Bion, W.R. (1963). *Elements of Psychoanalysis.* London: Karnac.
Frontline. (2014). *Secret State of North Korea.* PBS, January 14.
Green, A. (1999). *The Work of the Negative.* London: Free Association.
Hegel, G.W.F. (2003). *The Phenomenology of Mind.* London: Dover.

Chapter 15

Treating the traumatized mind

Dissociation and psychoanalytic technique

Michael J. Diamond[1]

Overview

Psychoanalysis has until very recently neglected the salience of *dissociation*. Consequently, the trauma field has been essentially relinquished to trauma theorists who tend to lack an understanding of dynamic unconscious processes that entail conflict, fantasy and actively motivated defenses. In order to offer a contemporary psychoanalytic perspective on treating the traumatized mind, I begin by noting that psychoanalysis had essentially replaced dissociation with repression, before clarifying how primary and secondary dissociation operate to attack linkages and disrupt symbolization.

In proposing to treat the "traumatized" psyche, both a repression-based model of mental functioning and one that incorporates dissociatively produced segregated units of experiencing are required. Moreover, whether trauma is acute or cumulative, child- or adult-onset, suffered at the hands of another or due to one one's own actions taken, the analyst must persistently analyze negative transferences as well as unconscious fantasies occurring both prior and subsequent to *the* trauma. This requires gearing treatment toward re-establishing symbolic capacities that dissociation disrupts and weakens. This chapter attempts to make these ideas clearer.

Psychoanalytic theorizing of trauma: an historical perspective

Recall that psychoanalysis emerged from Breuer and Freud's (1893) observation that the major reactive mechanism to trauma is, "severely paralysing affect … during a modified state of consciousness" (p. 110) that can only be introduced into normal consciousness through *speech*. Four years prior, Pierre Janet (1889) similarly described unconscious automatic activity in response to trauma. Both works agreed that dissociation involves consciousness splitting designed to exclude unpleasant memories or ideas (Gullestad, 2005). However, Freud stressed a dynamic defense (subsumed under repression) originating from internal *conflict*, whereas Janet focused on *deficit* produced by disorganized cognitive processing that he erroneously interpreted as the result of *passive* constitutional weakness.

The two soon became bitter rivals, with psychoanalysis starkly opposing the French view of psychopathology. Freud essentially erased "Janet's memory" (Ellenberger, 1970, p. 409; see also Makari, 2008) by replacing dissociation with the new concept of repression (while ingeniously incorporating its consciousness-splitting aspect) and calling his system "psycho-analysis" versus Janet's "psychological analysis". As Bromberg (1995) put it, "the restless ghost of Pierre Janet … [was] banished from the castle by Sigmund Freud" (p. 189).

Freud's failure to conceive of dissociation as autohypnotic-like yet resulting from an *active* motivated defense has been termed his "primal category mistake", one in which dissociation was omitted from the "venerable 'list' of psychoanalytic defense mechanisms" (O'Neil, 2018, pp. 262, 267). Consequently, whereas psychoanalysis emphasizes unconscious conflict and complex internal object relations, dissociative mental states have been largely overlooked and their "significance … [in]adequately addressed" (Bohleber, 2010, p. 131).

Psychoanalysis may have been set back following the Freud–Janet split by disregarding the traumatic reality of sexual abuse and incest as well as dissociation per se for many reasons—including clinical, methodological and identity politics. In fact, until recently, psychoanalysts have considered dissociation as "unsavoury" (Chase, 1991). Perhaps, as Alan Spivak (2005) suggests, "professional guilt" stemming from a long history of misunderstanding the "reality" of sexual abuse may have led to a compensatory over-focus on one end of the pendulum—namely, a perspective on trauma where the patient is more simply a passive "victim" of external reality (see also Spivak, this volume). Moreover, dissociation, if discussed at all, has been reduced to an automatic, psychobiologic response to overwhelming excitation. Unfortunately, and in contrast, trauma theorists retain interest in dissociative processes more mechanistically while largely excluding the dynamic unconscious so that the "who" or agent that decides to dissociate is largely omitted (Gullestad, 2005).

Despite its disappearance from psychoanalytic vocabulary, the phenomenon of dissociation and related autohypnotically fueled, defensive altered states of consciousness, with their segregated units of experience, remain unmistakable. Within psychoanalysis, consider Fairbairn's concept of *endopsychic ego structures*, Klein's *splitting of the self*, Federn's *ego states*, and Kohut's *self states*. Meanwhile, theorizing about trauma has continued to develop (notwithstanding dissociation's de-emphasis). For instance, Freud privileged pathological, primary process ego functioning and an object relations-based deficiency in protective shielding that accesses primal repression (1913, 1915, 1923). Ferenczi (1933), Fairbairn (1952 [1943]), Balint (1969), Winnicott (1974) and Khan (1974) furthered the view that the relationship with the object is the traumatogenic factor. Neo-Freudians, including Fenichel (1945) and subsequently Rothstein (1986), Shengold (1989) and Sugarman (1994), focused on ego regression to passive coping mechanisms, as well as libidinization of traumatic repetition that furthers sadomasochistic object relations. Meanwhile, North American interpersonal/relational theorists, particularly Bromberg (1991; 1995; 1998), Davies and Frawley (1994) and Stern (1997), have drawn on attachment and trauma theory to afford dissociation special status—albeit while minimizing its relationship to unconscious fantasy, impulse and conflict.

Though I welcome dissociation's return to the dialogue on both clinical and theoretical grounds, unfortunately, in a *pars pro toto* canard, several essential tenets of unconscious mental processing pertaining to primitive, endogenous fantasy and conflict have been *replaced* rather than *supplemented* by more mechanistic ideas pertaining to the revival of intolerable experience. Regrettably, many relational analysts reductively locate drive theory and object relations in opposition to the *relational turn* (e.g., Boulanger, 2007). Consequently, polarizing splits between various psychoanalytic camps are perpetuated, and useful technical ideas more closely aligned with trauma theory remain detached from indispensable, foundational psychoanalytic understandings that have been misconceived and reductively associated with Freud's renunciation of the so-called seduction theory (Gullestad, 2005; see also Bohleber, 2010).

Despite an overly broad concept of trauma (and dissociation) that is evident today, external, traumatizing conditions, environmental object relational failures and identification-based internalizations remain central. The word *trauma* comes from the Greek word meaning "wound", itself derivative of "to pierce". Analysts concur that psychic trauma always involves a "breach", a *too muchness* signified by its intensity and an incapacity to respond adequately, which produces mental upheaval with lasting consequences to the ego's construction of *meaning* (Shengold, 1989; Bohleber, 2010; see also Freud, 1920). Events are made traumatic by a specific interaction—namely, a "sudden and brutal encounter between an unconscious fantasy and external reality" (Bokanowski, 2005, p. 256). Such unconscious fantasies may include the illusion of complete security, blessedness and normal (healthy) omnipotence. Moreover, this interaction between the psyche and the environment is apparent in psychoanalytic work with *cumulative trauma* (Khan), *strain trauma* (Kris, Sandler), *silent trauma* (Hoffer) and *deprivation trauma* (Bowlby).

Nonetheless, as I have noted, the focus on unconscious fantasies and libidinal wishes has all but been *replaced* rather than more usefully *supplemented by* privileging trauma's quantitative impact on ego functioning and object relational failures in appropriate responsivity (e.g., the "negative" or absent external object). In sum, this *pars pro toto* fallacy continues to restrict our work and the *active agent*—the "I" doing the dissociating—is typically omitted. Thus, I maintain that a clinically based, dynamic tripod of analytic metapsychology grounded in *economic, topographical/structural conflict* and *object relational* understandings—what I think of as *the triadic nature of trauma* that incorporates dissociation—is necessary to treat trauma psychoanalytically.

Trauma and dissociation: representation, unconscious fantasy, conflict and internal objects

Reducing dissociation solely to a psychobiological, "shut-down" mechanism restricts work in the transference–countertransference field. It bears repeating then that trauma *always* reflects an interaction with the pre-existing, overdetermined internal world constructed in accordance with unconscious fantasies that are antecedent to, simultaneous with and/or subsequent to single-incident as well as cumulative trauma. Because cognitive functioning, including symbolization, thinking and integration, is compromised or suspended during traumatic experiences, unconscious fantasies—as well as archaic fantasy structures established during or soon after massive trauma (particularly in infancy or early childhood)—are less likely to be verbally represented and are typically more weakly symbolized (Rosenbaum & Vavrin, 2007).

Analytic treatment is particularly challenging because unconscious conflict and fantasy in traumatized patients is often more difficult to access because traditional interpretive methods primarily rely on freely associative, verbalizable material, whereas archaic fantasy structures associated with the trauma tend to be acted out nonverbally, often in the patient–analyst relationship (Vavrin, 2003). Consequently, as I will further elucidate, the nature and function of dissociation must be incorporated, requiring time and considerable effort until the secondary dissociative defenses alive in the transference are interpretively contained. The eventual pay-off is that unconscious fantasy and conflict-laden material become associatively linked to the primary dissociative mechanisms.

Dissociation

Winnicott (1945) was among the first neo-Freudians to posit that dissociation is a healthy, natural capacity—a "queer kind of truth" (1974, p. 105)—as well as a defensive response to trauma. He viewed dissociation as a natural capacity that precedes defensive repression and, like Bromberg, he believed that unlinked dissociated states lie at the root of all self-experience (see Goldman, 2012; 2013). Consequently, not all dissociations are indicative of psychopathology (though they may be defensively motivated), and human beings seem to have an innate capacity to become dissociatively absorbed for creatively adaptive purposes as well as for self-protective, defensive ones.

Adaptive, healthy dissociative experience is evident, for instance, in splits between the observing ego and the experiencing ego, splits that are part of the analyst's "therapeutic dissociations" (Sterba, 1934). Similarly, quotidian dissociative experience resting on autohypnotic ability (Butler, 2006) is apparent when we engage in creatively imaginative play; in states of artistic immersion; when we are absorbed in reading, music, cinema or theater; when we watch or play sports; in spiritual experiences, intoxicated states, hypnosis or "highway hypnosis" while driving; and in other consciousness-altering experiences or states of mind (Hilgard, 1977).

The link between severe trauma and dissociation is generally well established (Hilgard, 1977; van der Kolk, 1986; 2006; Diamond, 1997; 2018; Bohleber, 2010). More extreme dissociative experience tends to remain unsymbolized in thought and language, "cut off from authentic human relatedness" (Bromberg, 1991, pp. 405–6) and generating an "unconscious refusal to be curious" (Stern, 1997, p. 6). Unlike repression, dissociation does *not* produce a forgetting of threatening mental content, but instead keeps them segregated and partly available *only in specific states of mind* by severing ties between linked self-state processes. Analysts, beginning with Freud, who are familiar with hypnosis can appreciate that these altered self-states can be more easily activated through hypnotic, imagistic and bodily-based interventions.

It is important, however, to distinguish *primary dissociation* from *secondary dissociation*, though in their defensive functioning, both these phenomena express an overwhelmed ego's protective and often quite adaptive altered state. Consequently, despite operating under conditions of failure of synthesis and integration, dissociation forecloses psychic contents and severs connections between mental contents to modulate unbearable internal states (particularly intense impulses and emotions) and thereby salvage minimally needed mental functioning (Gullestad 2005; see also Janet, 1889; Davies & Frawley, 1994).

In *primary dissociation*, overwhelmingly traumatic events activate the individual's annihilation anxieties—an "original experience of primitive agony" (Winnicott, 1974, p. 105)—so that unconscious, protective autoregulation keeps psychic experiences separated from consciousness while obliterating the sense of personal agency. An experienced "unbearableness" causes the "I" to leave the scene (in a hypnoid state) in order to maintain personhood or sanity in the face of breakdown (Diamond, 1997; see also Winnicott, 1974; Goldman, 2012).

In contrast, *secondary dissociation*, as often experienced in the analytic setting, reflects a motivated defensive operation originating in unconscious internal conflict. Secondary dissociation requires interpretive acumen inasmuch as both passive and active ego defenses are in play. The physiological effects are less intense than in primary dissociation, yet there is a persistence of the defense of turning away from threatening stimuli (such as the analyst in the negative transference). Such dissociation becomes structurally organized in complex character patterns originating in intrapsychic conflict—for example, in dissociative identity disorders (e.g., multiple personality) and those dissociative defensive structures evident in eating and addictive disorders, psychosomatic reactions, borderline personality disorders, schizoid states and posttraumatic stress disorders.

Distinguishing between primary and secondary dissociation, as well as between dissociation and repression, is far less clear-cut in treatment because dissociative processes inevitably connect themselves to other defensive maneuvers. Patients utilize both secondary dissociation and repression against any undesirable intrapsychic material (Gullestad, 2005; Bohleber, 2010), and diminution in the sense of *I-ness* often reflects dissociative mechanisms having become secondarily linked with conflictual material. Nonetheless, I propose that in order to help recover the patient's lost sense of agency the analyst must first carefully validate the psychic state associated with annihilating anxieties *prior to* interpreting the conflictual fantasies and object representations. For instance, merely interpreting a patient's "attacks on linking" (Bion, 1962) cannot do justice to the horrendously fragmenting states of mind that have become linked to seemingly more straightforward, conflict-based compromise formations.

Memory and representation

Because trauma overwhelms memory's integrative functioning and alters normative linking among memory systems (Diamond, 1997; Bohleber, 2010; see also Schacter, 1996), the continuity of time is significantly disrupted. Rather than flowing continuously, the patient's sense of time seems stuck in a permanent "now"—the Lacanian "real"—like a succession of dangerous, jagged peaks (Scarfone, 2006). In Lacanian terms, what has not been allowed symbolic expression reappears in reality in the form of a hallucination (Lacan, 1966).

Through dissociated self states, traumatic memories tend to remain encapsulated and isolated from the remaining flow of affectively laden, associative linkages. Consequently, such memories are subject to little or no revision by present circumstances, although they are generally preserved with considerable precision (not necessarily accuracy) in the unconscious. In addition, the patient's traumatic experience of *primitive agony* (Ferenczi, 1933), *mental disaster* or *breakdown* (Winnicott, 1974) or *internal catastrophe* (Bion, 1992), as well as the accompanying unconscious fantasies, remains split off and psychically undigested (cf. Bion, 1962).

Trauma in the analytic situation

In the analytic situation, we see that the patient's *experience of trauma* depends on *what is made of* the impinging external events and corresponding endogenous, often predetermined stimulation. Traumatized patients often reveal how their psychic functioning is undone by self-protective dissociative mechanisms, which, as Freud (1920) argued in *Beyond the Pleasure Principle*, restores pleasure principle functioning while disrupting the continuity of time and identity as well as weakening symbolization (Shengold, 1989; Bohleber, 2010). Potentially representable experience remains unintegrated, timeless and ego alien because the dissociated "raw data" stored as traumatic memory and left devoid of symbolism, yet often rendered in somatic symptoms, cannot undergo further mental processing (Bokanowski, 2005).

Consequently, the absence or unknown source of pain requires transformation into a psychic presence through the analyst's interpretively providing meaning (McDougall, 1974; Aisenstein, 2006)—hence, when dissociative experience is put into words and images, forgetting through the work of *repression* can occur. This is easier said than done, however, because the disruptions in memory and representational functioning often force the analyst to "suffer with" the patient's terrified states of mind and to endure deadening dissociative defensive operations before utilizing representational interventions. *Vicarious traumatization* experienced by the analyst often ensues, and may become a necessary therapeutic tool for representing and interpreting the meaning that has been unconsciously repudiated (Diamond, 2014; 2018). As I attempt to clarify next, successful treatment often rests on gradually developing the ego's capacity to represent such encrypted psychic experiences and to mentally process unbearable anxieties and psychic pain (Birksted-Breen et al., 2010).

Analytic technique amid dissociative functioning

The analyst must discern not only how the traumatization is represented—despite how tenuously its representational elements are connected to early trauma—but also how *accessible* the fragments of traumatic memory, affect and fantasy are to the patient's consciousness and associative processes. Consequently, the analyst needs to determine what sort of mind is being dealt with at any point—a mind capable of imaginative and metaphorical thinking, or perhaps a more somatically based one with a more limited capacity for symbol formation.

Because a central role is played by the actuality of trauma—namely, vital memories and experiences that remain segregated and are yet to be creatively imagined and represented—I will briefly consider the clinical challenges that arise when trauma does not yet belong to the sphere of repression but instead is stored in the body. The key issue is how to transform these somatic memory traces into more "normal" memory—to find ways of translating the unrepresentable and making it psychically *figurable* (Botella & Botella, 2005; Civitarese, 2013).

This process typically commences when the analyst can address the trauma's impact on the patient's symbolizing capacities. Whether it is assumed that symbolization is disrupted by means of a deficiency in psychic structure or as a product of underlying conflict and unconscious fantasy, I contend that representation is best understood as occurring in gradients—ranging from very weak, bodily-based forms to stronger ones that are verbally and imaginatively encoded. Consequently, I find a *dual-track* technical approach advantageous, one that entails both *archeological* and *transformational* ways of working (Levine, 2012). The first of these addresses well-represented and symbolically invested psychic elements tangled in conflict; and the second is required to translate the semiotic, pre-representational and sensual into the symbolic realm.

Archeological work requires an investigative analytic attitude, with a more knowing analyst serving to interpret the patient's repressed unconscious in order to discern concealed meaning apropos conflict pathology. *Transformational* work, on the other hand, requires an affirmative mode to establish meaning (Killingmo, 1989; 2006), and here the analyst is more of an "engaged witness to the 'queer truth' of dissociated experience" (Goldman, 2016, p. 105). Most analyses with traumatized patients are characterized by oscillations between both these modes, and the central technical issue is the analyst's ability to discover what kind of mind the patient is operating from and to tailor his interventions accordingly.

To disentangle the actuality of the trauma (i.e., traumatic "reality") from unconscious conflict and fantasy, the patient needs to experience the analyst's sufficient validation of the traumatic events themselves. This entails discovering the "reality" of the trauma and its associated effects, however approximate. Of course, working with the patient's psychic reality in relation to actual, historic reality is a complex matter (see Diamond, 1997); at the very least, doing so requires the analyst to "believe skeptically and doubt empathically" (Brenneis, 1994, p. 1050). Nonetheless, validation in the realm of "actual" trauma helps the dissociative, traumatized patient become sufficiently available to the recognition and analysis of secondary revisions via unconscious fantasies, conflictual affects and defensive constructions (often involving introjective and projective punitive impulses and guilty feelings). Otherwise, the danger of iatrogenic retraumatization remains in the form of repeating the traumatic impact of nonrecognition by the "absent" ("negative") caregiving object (Ferenczi, 1933).

The variously traumatized analyst becomes "impregnated" by turbulent affect (McDougall, 1978). In this charged atmosphere of projective identification with the patient's unsymbolized terrors and unbearable states of falling apart, the analyst—despite feeling confused, overwhelmed, helpless, enraged, betrayed, guilty, powerfully protective and driven to act—must discern the patient's negative transferences, which often remain disguised by compliant and/or defiant character modes (Diamond, 1997). Given the analyst's likelihood of "falling ill" with the ailment affecting the patient (Borgogno, 2014), there is a high potential for the analyst to *enact*—and particularly to assume a masochistic or sadistic stance in identifying with the patient's inner objects rather than recovering in order to contain and subsequently to interpretively represent.

When *secondary dissociation* appears—at times as an extremely varied, "weird" scenario, and at other times in more subtle ways (Diamond, 1997; Gullestad, 2005)—the analyst must both appreciate its function as a motivated defense implying an active, albeit unconscious strategic agent, *and* yet still recognize it as something that just "happens" to the passively experiencing patient through repetition compulsion. However, like other forms of repetition compulsion, secondary dissociation expresses an archaic effort at mastery, which in the analyst's presence represents an active attempt to find in the analyst a containing object capable of making sense of what has remained weakly symbolized.

In short, the analyst's recognition, containment and skillful interpretive work allows the dissociated aspects of the patient that cannot yet speak—the dissociated *not me* state possessing the patient—to be experienced as a presence that the patient is able to own and thus to represent (initially, together with the analyst). The patient's unconscious fantasies and conflicts often become more accessible when the analyst, through reconstruction, labels (secondarily) dissociative-based experience as *traumatic* and affirmatively links it to the here-and-now transference (Killingmo, 2006). The analyst accomplishes this by interpreting what may be occurring "at the same time and on another level" (Grotstein, 2009). The following clinical material should make this evident.

Clinical vignette

A brief analytic vignette with Ms. A, an adult woman severely traumatized by chronic early childhood abuse, is illustrative. (NB: This case is discussed in greater detail both in Diamond, 1997 and Diamond, 2018.) Following successful interpretive work that enabled her to experience me as "accepting" her desires and unconscious fantasies to be "loved" by her sexually abusive father by sitting on his lap and receiving his undivided attention, Ms. A abruptly began to dissociate in the session. My interpretive labeling of what she experienced passively could occur only after a considerable period during which I felt increasingly helpless, particularly when she seemed to "disappear" in an eerie fashion (thus enacting a "queer kind of truth"), as she did during frequent dissociative episodes. These episodes manifested in abrupt shifts in Ms. A's consciousness, which at this time took the form of her looking at me in an ominous manner and then stroking what she referred to as the "mask" that had befallen her face. In time, when she was able to verbalize her experience, she described herself as "dissolving and spacing out" and then became catatonic, as if paralyzed.

Though feeling "impregnated" by disturbing, turbulent affect, I eventually recovered my ability to think. I said to her:

> You are experiencing my recent comment that made you feel "loved" in a way that caused you to re-live how you felt with your father [the abuser] and so your "traumatized mind" seems to take you over again.

She stared ahead as I continued:

> This paralyzed state originally occurred when you felt so overwhelmed and helpless with no one around who was able to help you make sense of what was happening to you. You felt flooded by what was going on inside and around you and so, then like now, you try to escape from yourself. It seems there is no other way to protect yourself and survive except by "spacing out" and putting on a mask that makes you feel invulnerable to physical pain and unbearable thoughts and feelings.

As she began to tear up and make eye contact with me, she said:

> But *there is* no other way.

Recognizing the return of her symbolizing "agent", I resumed (by interpreting the secondary dissociation and the accompanying conflict and preconscious fantasy):

> It seems that when your positive feelings toward me emerge, you suddenly anticipate that my being "nice" will lead to my betraying you. The conflict you experience feels unbearable because you experience your desire to feel loved and tenderly connected; and yet you imagine that I will soon hurt you and that you'll be helpless. You start to re-live feeling all alone once again with excruciating terror, guilt, anger and, as we've discussed, excitement. And so, you make your experience with me disappear into your "spaced-out" mask the way you so often do.

Brief discussion and conclusion

Such interpretive-based labeling, linked to the trauma that has remained frozen in time, helps create sufficient distance in the patient's mind so that the reestablishment of symbolizing abilities can begin. In short, the intersubjective space previously compromised (and largely foreclosed) after massive psychic trauma can be recreated. The dead space that had been frozen in time is recoverable and can be brought to life in the transference. In this respect, the third that was dead is brought back through a form of *analytic witnessing* (Gerson, 2009), and thus unconscious conflicts and fantasies can then be interpreted in the "traumatic" transference.

The challenge in working with a traumatized psyche lies in the analyst's skills and abilities in validating the actuality of the trauma and its object relational failures while finding ways to access and interpret the intrapsychic fantasies, constructions and identifications that have impacted the experiencing of trauma. The analyst's witnessing, experiencing and suffering, as well as his articulation of the dissociated experience in analytic space, enable the *now-ness* of unconscious, actual (traumatized) time to become partially transferred into psychic representation. As a result, the movement into present tense permits the trauma to begin its entry into chronological time, and thus an analytic transformation to begin.

Note

1 Portions of this chapter were originally presented as an invited presentation for the CIPS/NAPsaC Clinical Conference on "Trauma, Destruction and Transformative Potential" held in New York City, May 2014.

References

Aisenstein, M. (2006). The indissociable unity of psyche and soma: A view from the Paris Psychosomatic School. *International Journal of Psychoanalysis*, 87: 667–680.

Balint, M. (1969). Trauma and object relationship. *International Journal of Psychoanalysis*, 50: 429–435.

Bion, W.R. (1962). The psycho-analytic study of thinking: II. A theory of thinking. *International Journal of Psychoanalysis*, 43: 306–310.

Bion, W.R. (1992). *Cogitations*. London: Karnac.

Birksted-Breen, D., Flanders, S. & Gibeault, A. (2010). *Reading French Psychoanalysis*. London: Routledge.

Bohleber, W. (2010). *Destructiveness, Intersubjectivity, and Trauma: The Identity Crisis of Modern Psychoanalysis*. London: Karnac.

Bokanowski, T. (2005). Variations on the concept of traumatism: Traumatism, traumatic, trauma. *International Journal of Psychoanalysis*, 86: 251–265.

Borgogno, F. (2014). "Coming from afar" and "temporarily becoming the patient without knowing it": Two necessary analytic conditions according to Ferenczi's later thought. *American Journal of Psychoanalysis*, 74: 302–312.

Botella, C. & Botella, S. (2005). *The Work of Psychic Figurability: Mental States without Representation*. Hove, New York, NY: Brunner Routledge.

Boulanger, G. (2007). *Wounded By Reality: Understanding and Treating Adult Onset Trauma*. Mahwah, NJ: Analytic Press.

Brenneis, C.B. (1994). Belief and suggestion in the recovery of memories of childhood sexual abuse. *Journal of the American Psychoanalytic Association*, 42: 1027–1053.

Breuer, J. & Freud, S. (1893). On the psychical mechanism of hysterical phenomena: Preliminary communication. *Standard Edition 2*: 3–17. London: Hogarth Press.

Bromberg, P.M. (1991). On knowing one's patient inside out: The aesthetics of unconscious communication. *Psychoanalytic Dialogues*, 1: 399–422.

Bromberg, P.M. (1995). Psychoanalysis, dissociation, and personality organization. *Standing in the Spaces: Essays on Clinical Process, Trauma, and Dissociation*. Hillsdale, NJ: Analytic Press, 1998, 189–294.

Bromberg, P.M. (1998). *Standing in the Spaces: Essays on Clinical Process, Trauma, and Dissociation*. Hillsdale, NJ: Analytic Press.

Butler, L.D. (2006). Normative dissociation. *Psychiatric Clinics of North America*, 29: 45–62.

Chase, J.S. (1991). Hypnosis revisited: Toward an integrated approach. *International Review of Psycho-Analysis*, 18: 513–526.

Civitarese, G. (2013). *The Violence of Emotions: Bion and Post-Bionian Psychoanalysis*. London: Routledge.
Davies, J.M. & Frawley, M.G. (1994). *Treating the Adult Survivor of Childhood Sexual Abuse: A Psychoanalytic Perspective*. New York: Basic Books.
Diamond, M.J. (1997). The unbearable agony of being: Interpreting tormented states of mind in the psychoanalysis of sexually traumatized patients. *Bulletin of the Menninger Clinic*, 61: 495–519.
Diamond, M.J. (2014). Analytic mind use and interpsychic communication: Driving force in analytic technique, pathway to unconscious mental life. *Psychoanalytic Quarterly*, 83: 525–563.
Diamond, M.J. (2018). The return of the repressed: Dissociation, metapsychology, and the psychoanalysis of the traumatized mind. Unpublished paper.
Ellenberger, H.F. (1970). *The Discovery of the Unconscious*. New York: Basic Books.
Fairbairn, W.R.D. (1952). The repression and the return of bad objects (with special reference to the "war neuroses"). *Psychoanalytic Studies of the Personality*. London: Tavistock, 59–81). (Original work published 1943).
Fenichel, O. (1945). *Psychoanalytic Theory of Neurosis, Volume I*. New York: Norton.
Ferenczi, S. (1933). Confusion of tongues between adults and the child. *International Journal of Psychoanalysis*, 30: 225–230.
Freud, S. (1913). On psycho-analysis. *Standard Edition 12*: 205–213. London: Hogarth Press.
Freud, S. (1915). Repression. *Standard Edition 14*: 141–158. London: Hogarth Press.
Freud, S. (1918). From the history of an infantile neurosis. *Standard Edition 17*, 3–124. London: Hogarth Press.
Freud, S. (1920). Beyond the pleasure principle. *Standard Edition 18*: 7–64. London: Hogarth Press.
Freud, S. (1923). The ego and the id. *Standard Edition 19*: 12–68. London: Hogarth Press.
Gerson, S. (2009). When the third is dead: Memory, mourning, and witnessing in the aftermath of the Holocaust. *International Journal of Psychoanalysis*, 90: 1341–1357.
Goldman, D. (2012). Weaving with the world: Winnicott's reimagining of reality, *Psychoanalytic Quarterly*, 81: 1–24.
Goldman, D. (2013). Vital sparks and the form of things unknown. *Psychoanalytic Inquiry*, 33: 3–20.
Goldman, D. (2016). "A queer kind of truth": Winnicott and the uses of dissociation. *The Dissociative Mind in Psychoanalysis: Understanding and Working with Trauma*, E.F. Howell & S. Itzkowitz (eds.). New York: Routledge, 97–106.
Grotstein, J.S. (2009). *"…But at the Same Time and On Another Level…". Vols. 1 & 2*. London: Karnac.
Gullestad, S.E. (2005). Who is "who" in dissociation? A plea for psychodynamics in a time of trauma. *International Journal of Psychoanalysis*, 86: 639–656.
Hilgard, E.R. (1977). *Divided Consciousness: Multiple Controls in Human Thought and Action*. New York: Wiley.
Janet, P. (1889). *L'Automatisme Psychologique*. Paris: Felix Alcan.
Killingmo, B. (1989). Conflict and deficit: Implications for technique. *International Journal of Psychoanalysis*, 70: 65–79.
Killingmo, B. (2006). A plea for affirmation relating to states of unmentalised affects. *Scandinavian Psychoanalytic Review*, 29: 13–21.

Lacan, J. (1966). *Écrits: The First Complete Edition in English*, trans. B. Fink. New York: Norton, 2006.
Levine, H.B. (2012). The colourless canvas: Representation, therapeutic action and the creation of mind. *International Journal of Psychoanalysis*, 93: 607–629.
Makari, G. (2008). *Revolution in Mind: The Creation of Psychoanalysis.* New York: Harper.
McDougall, J. (1974). The psychosoma and the psychoanalytic process. *International Review of Psychoanalysis*, 1: 437–459.
McDougall, J. (1978). Primitive communication and the use of countertransference: Reflections on early psychic trauma and its transference effects. *Contemporary Psychoanalysis*, 14: 173–209.
O'Neil, J.A. (2018). Hypnosis and psychoanalysis: Toward undoing Freud's primal category mistake. *American Journal of Clinical Hypnosis*, 60: 262–278.
Rosenbaum, B. & Vavrin, S. (2007). The influence of extreme traumatization on the body, mind and social relations. *International Journal of Psychoanalysis*, 88: 1527–1542.
Rothstein, A. (1986). *The Reconstruction of Trauma: Its Significance in Clinical Work.* Madison, CT: International Universities Press.
Scarfone, D. (2006). A matter of time and the production of the past. *Psychoanalytic Quarterly*, 75: 807–834.
Schacter, D.L. (1996). *Searching For Memory: The Brain, the Mind, and the Past.* New York: Basic Books.
Shengold, L. (1989). *Soul Murder.* New Haven, CT: Yale University Press.
Spivak, A.P. (2005). The central role of unconscious fantasy in the analysis of child abuse trauma. Paper presented at the 44th International Psychoanalytical Association Congress, Rio de Janeiro, Brazil.
Sterba, R. (1934). The fate of the ego in analytic therapy. *International Journal of Psychoanalysis*, 15: 117–126.
Stern, D.B. (1997). *Unformulated Experience: From Dissociation to Imagination in Psychoanalysis.* Hillsdale, NJ: Analytic Press.
Sugarman, A. (1994). *Victims of Abuse: The Emotional Impact of Child and Adult Trauma.* Madison, CT: International Universities Press.
Van der Kolk, B.A. (1986). *Psychological Trauma.* Washington, DC: American Psychiatric Press.
Van der Kolk, B.A. (2006). Clinical implications of neuroscience research in PTSD. *Annual New York Academy of Sciences*, 1071: 277–293.
Vavrin, S. (2003). *Mental Survival Strategies after Extreme Traumatization.* Copenhagen: Multivers.
Winnicott, D.W. (1945). Primitive emotional development. *International Journal of Psychoanalysis*, 26: 137–143.
Winnicott, D.W. (1974). Fear of breakdown. *International Review of Psychoanalysis*, 1: 103–107.

Chapter 16

The central role of unconscious fantasy in the analysis of child abuse trauma

Alan P. Spivak

Introduction

This contribution addresses an imbalance that has evolved in the literature of child abuse trauma downplaying the role of fantasy that predates the abuse.[1] By contrast, I argue below that a child's reactions to sexual abuse—including symptoms, memories, fantasies and dissociated states of mind that postdate the trauma—are pivotally forged by unconscious erotic and aggressive fantasies that he/she imports to the trauma from earlier phases of development, which may themselves have been problematic for the child's growth trajectory. These fantasies stamp incidents of sexual trauma with multiple meanings that, often, are quite primitive and terrifying. The analysis of these fantasies as they emerge in psychoanalytic transferences of adults can:

1 Give access to repressed and dissociated memories of the trauma.
2 Elucidate multiple meanings that have been encoded into the memories.
3 Facilitate the integration of the post-abuse sequelae into the psychic life of the analysand.
4 Provide access to repressed memories, introjects and non-sexual traumas from developmental periods preceding the abuse.
5 Enable vital transference resistances and enactments to be recognized and worked through.

After some preliminary remarks regarding the trend in the literature nearly to ignore drive-based fantasy that predates the trauma while privileging fantasy, symptoms and other sequelae that postdate it, I demonstrate my thesis with detailed material from a clinical case in which the analysand, as an oedipal age child, unconsciously construed sexual intimacies with her father to be the return of her own primitive sadistic and incorporative urges from earlier in her life that she had directed toward the body of a mother who was experienced by her as inconsistently available. In essence, through condensation and the law of talion, her father's intrusive fondling had become equated with her own oral longings toward her pre-oedipal mother. Consequently, the incest was experienced as a devouring encounter with a mother-father-monster who was cannibalizing her.

The gross failure of the father to resonate with the developmental needs of the young girl, including her need for boundaries, magnified exponentially the psychic disrepair of the earlier mother–daughter dyad. A second chance for the maternally deprived child, i.e., repair through father–daughter love, was squandered. Since her father's body was all too present and his emotional attunement absent, the girl's overtaxed defensive system fell back on desperate measures to stave off psychic collapse. Among these were splitting, dissociation and idealization.

I will illustrate with vignettes from two time frames within the analysis, corresponding to two developmental levels, pre-oedipal and oedipal, the use of an idealized-erotized transference for a dual purpose: 1. To help ward off unconscious terrifying primitive fantasies of invading the body of the early mother and stealing its life giving supplies; 2. To mask fragmented and dissociated memories of sexual intimacies with father. Additionally, I will demonstrate that erotic idealization within the transference can serve simultaneously as a resistance and as a temporarily adaptive mechanism by which a desperate woman can keep alive a tenuous hope for growth and repair through a connection with a transformational object (Bollas, 1987). Finally, I will highlight interpretations, and the analysand's responses to them, as she begins to come to terms with her core anxieties.

Background

Fantasy and trauma theory

Differing psychoanalytic theories share as common ground Freud's original notion that an adult's mental life is formed by the comingling of multiple events, external and psychic, across three time frames: the distant past of childhood, the more recent past, and the immediate present. Freud's theories of the psychoneuroses and of dreams draw heavily on this concept. A neurotic symptom, for example, derives its meaning from condensations of experience and fantasy over time. To understand a symptom, in its complexity, one must become familiar with its antecedents, internal and external, from all three time frames. Dreams, too, condense a childhood memory or fantasy, the day residue and the immediate need to sleep (Freud, 1900).

Theories of traumatic neuroses—Freud (1936), Fenichel (1937), Balint (1969), Blum (1987)—also give prominence to considerations of antecedent events over the three time frames. For example, a soldier in combat may develop a phobic symptom that, as a subsequent analysis reveals, condenses an unconscious conflict over separation from his mother of infancy (the distant past) that was reawakened when he was shipped overseas (the recent past) with hyper-awareness of his vulnerability to annihilation that was provoked by a bomb exploding near him and killing members of his squad (the immediate present). An analysis would ordinarily be considered incomplete if fantasies related to the separation conflict of childhood were not linked to an understanding of the trauma.

The omission of fantasy in child sexual abuse studies

When trauma theory is extended to child abuse considerations the notions of overdetermination and condensation of psychic events over time often lose their way, as investigators tend to focus more heavily on the psychic consequences of sexual abuse while minimizing the antecedent mental state of the child. This skewed emphasis has resulted in a literature that in many respects is quite illuminating. But, in giving short shrift to the antecedent mental life and the specific meanings it stamps on the trauma for a given child, the literature leans toward generalization and stereotypy. Usually, the clinical reports focus on the defensive measures a child employed to deal with the traumatic impact of severe overstimulation and aggression at the hands of an abusing adult. Chief among these are splitting, dissociation and identification with the aggressor. The aftermath of the trauma as reflected in subsequent symptomatology and character disturbances is also emphasized. The role played by parents is bifurcated: One parent is the seducer (abuser), the other is the abandoner. Subsequent guilt, aggression or masochism often is attributed routinely to identification with the abuser.

More recently many excellent studies have enlarged our understanding of dissociated and unformulated states. (See Diamond in this volume for detailed distinctions between primary dissociation, secondary dissociation and repression, and for his well-documented reminder of the importance of unconscious conflict impacting trauma.) Other excellent studies of dissociation include: Bohleber (2012), Bromberg (1998), Davies & Frawley (1994) and Gullestad (2005). Recent work with unformulated states includes: Botella & Botella (2005), Civitarese (2013), Levine (2012) and Stern (2003).

Even these newer studies tend to ignore or minimize in their clinical examples how the pre-existing state of mind of the child interprets the abuse. For example, identifications with bad objects from earlier in the developmental history, which co-determine how the child interpreted the traumatic experience, are often left out altogether, or are unelaborated in favor of an emphasis on identification with the abuser, which is a process that postdates the trauma. Family dynamics frequently are described in general terms, but their specific influence on the mind of the child during the abuse is often unmentioned. Bigras (1990), for example, coined the term "negative incest" to refer to the mother's failure to protect the child from the abuser. He suggests that maternal deprivation leaves a needy child ripe for seduction. While this is a fruitful generalization, Bigras does not go on to address the impact of the maternal failure on the child's specific interpretation of the abuse, i.e., he does not tell us what is going on unconsciously in the child's mind.

To summarize, the unconscious meaning which the child gives to its precocious sexual experience, that is, his/her construal of what is happening to him/her at the time of the abuse, usually is ignored. This meaning is, in turn, co-determined by his/her character structure, phase of development, family dynamics and internal object world—that is, by factors predating the abuse.

Particularly noteworthy in these reports is the neglect of drive-related unconscious fantasy constellations, which, as I will soon show, constitute templates—that is, psychic anlagen for the child's construal of what is happening to him/her during the trauma. The effect of this omission is to treat the mind of the child at the time of the abuse as if it were a tabula rasa which, not having a psychic context, can only react to the abuse rather reflexively, within a limited range of responses. This neglect of unconscious fantasy, a primary constituent of psychic reality, is in stark contrast to psychoanalytic case reports detailing other forms of psychopathology, including traumatic neuroses unrelated to sexual abuse.

One might speculate that professional guilt, stemming from a long history in psychoanalysis in which the reality of sexual abuse was understated, has driven analysts to focus now predominantly at the other end of the pendulum, where the patient is viewed singularly, and one-dimensionally, as a victim whose subsequent difficulties stem solely from external reality and whose libidinal and aggressive urges play a marginalized role in what makes the abuse traumatic for the child.

Fantasy in an integrated approach

In contrast to this longstanding trend in theorizing child sexual abuse, I am proposing that unconscious fantasies, condensed over time, stamp an incident of abuse with specific meaning(s). This formulation squares with writers such as Fairbairn (1943 [1952]), Balint (1969) and Schafer (1992), who from different theoretical perspectives also emphasize that to understand the effects of trauma one must consider the interaction of trauma with the pre-existing internal world of the child. From his object relational point of view, for example, Fairbairn stressed a person's need to depend on early objects. For him trauma such as child abuse is reacted to uniquely in accord with the status of the internal world of objects extant at the time. For an adult to remember being abused as a child is to risk the release of a bad object from the past and to suffer terrible separation anxiety.

Balint, who also favored an integrated approach, suggested bringing trauma theory into alignment with the structural theory by emphasizing the role of the early maternal relationship on the child's interpretation of the later trauma. "Dependent people, as is generally known, create intensely tempting situations for the release of suppressed drives" (1969, p. 432). Here Balint is referring to the drives of others. But he does not go on to show how dependency is represented psychically. Neither does he address the child's erotic and aggressive drives, as opposed to the abuser's, that co-determine the particular intrapsychic representation of the dependency. In other words, he stops short of addressing unconscious fantasy.

More recently Schafer, while discussing the interaction of internalization and projection, has remarked that:

> much more is involved in the analysand's suffering than having been victimized by her or his family's unmistakably cruel or otherwise disturbing exercises of power … it is likely to include the analysand's having become … either a seducer of sadism or, through identification, a ruthless wielder of power and a cruel victimizer of others, often in the most subtle way. (1992, pp. 128–129)

Schafer, too, is speaking exclusively to manifestations of post-traumatic phenomena.

An object relations perspective

The object relations model for understanding trauma that I am proposing here differs from notions of other investigators who define trauma in terms of Freud's (1936) economic model in which the ego is said to be exposed to stimulation which overwhelms and floods it. The formulation that I am advancing is compatible with Fairbairn's view of the release of bad objects. But, unlike Fairbairn's view, the bad object does not represent solely the qualities of the frustrating parent. It contains, as well, the original aggressiveness of the child's own oral incorporative and sadistic drives. In this respect my object relations model is closer to notions of Klein (1975) and Kernberg (1976).

The spectrum from collusion to aggression

Many accounts of child abuse focus on extremely aggressive, even violent, actions of an aggressor toward a child who is helpless to do anything but endure her plight, that is, to do whatever she can to physically and psychically survive. Splitting, dissociation and identification with the aggressor are measures desperately taken to make survival possible, since physical fight or flight are not options. It is generally recognized, however, that abusers' aggressiveness exists along a wide spectrum. At one end of the continuum overt aggressiveness is minimal in relation to gentle seductiveness (see Gullestad, 2005). To a child in need of tender relatedness, particularly to one who has been significantly deprived of it, gentle erotic contact may at first be welcomed as it is misunderstood by the young mind as finally receiving what is missing and longed for. These cases in particular afford one the opportunity to observe in the transference a child's enactment of unconscious fantasy and unfulfilled desire toward an early maternal object that is carried forward to a later object, maternal or paternal, who is willing to join her in violating the incest taboo. In these instances, from the child's perspective, the abuser's abuse, the trauma, may be less the intrusion of aggressive or violent sexuality as much as a failure in boundary setting and/or in exposing the child, eventually, to incidents of excruciatingly humiliating rejection when he has had enough of her. (This will be illustrated shortly in the case presented below.)

Analysis versus absolution

The vital importance to an analysand of her analyst acknowledging and accepting her "willing" participation in seductive instances of abuse has been brought home to me in recent years by female patients who told of their despair and increase in feelings of guilt when previous therapists allegedly had taken an accusatory stance toward the abuser while turning a blind eye to aspects of the erotic contact which they had experienced as pleasurable and comforting. Ironically, it seems that, when an analyst, in a well-meaning but authoritarian stance, attempts to absolve a patient of the "sin" of incest by encouraging her to forgive herself and blame the abuser, the patient hears only that the analyst cannot accept her willing participation and concludes that she is a sinner. It would seem that her harsh superego has a louder voice than that of her gentle analyst. By contrast, when the analyst restricts himself to nonjudgmental exploration of the patient's fantasies of the erotic contact, including its dual purpose in maintaining hope and fending off despair, she may gradually come to accept and integrate the collusive participation. In other words, she gradually may be able to enter a state of mind in which she can work through the guilt and shame associated with it.

A case of child sexual abuse

In vignettes from two time frames of an analysis reflecting two developmental levels, oedipal and pre-oedipal, I will illustrate a woman's use of an idealized-erotized transference to ward off recognition of terrifying primitive erotic and aggressive fantasies.[2] I will show that her recovery by interpretation led to fragmented memories of a sexual collusion with her father. The erotic idealization, additionally, will be shown to be more than simply a resistance. It must also be appreciated as an adaptive mechanism by which a desperate woman could keep alive a tenuous hope for growth and repair through a connection with the analyst who serves as a transformational object (Bollas, 1987).

The patient, Beverly—a bright, 47-year-old married woman who was accomplished in her profession—had been in analysis five times per week for four years. Of medium height and with blonde hair, her speech was colored with the words and enunciations of a younger, less educated person. She is a physical therapist with a successful practice. Married for 25 years to an accountant, she has 4 children (2 boys and 2 girls) ranging from 14 to 22. Her presenting complaints were: 1. a general lack of confidence; 2. anxiety, approaching panic, when she taught or lectured; 3. chronic bodily tenseness; and 4. a distaste for, and avoidance of, sexual intercourse with her husband.

History

This brief history emerged gradually through the first several months of the analysis, and was offered by the patient quite spontaneously. Beverly is the fifth of five children, Jewish, born and reared in Canada. Her mother and father fought frequently, and were remembered as hating each other. Mother was tired and ill throughout most of Beverly's childhood. Beverly held two views of herself: On the one hand, she was a child whose presence and exuberance burdened her often exhausted mother; on the other, she was the gleam in her mother's eye, when her mother had the energy to gleam. Mother worked hard with household chores during the day, but was experienced as too busy to spend much time with Beverly. She napped often, leaving Beverly alone to feel abandoned. When she was awake, Beverly often followed mother from room to room as she cleaned the house. Beverly tried to fill lonely hours by playing with her two-year older sister and her friends, but she was often rebuffed. Her father was seen as stubborn, irritable and given to impulsive rages that terrified her. Father, sister and even mother mocked her for "always wanting too much and never being satisfied".

Process

An idealized transference

In the transference I quickly became idealized: I was termed "bright", "empathic", "sensitive", "a really nice person". Beverly, for her part, seemed to assign herself the role of an awkward, compliant, non-complaining child-woman. She greatly looked forward to her analytic hours, becoming slightly depressed and anxious on Friday afternoons as she anticipated the weekend break. She eagerly awaited the Monday hour, and although she functioned well in her professional and family responsibilities over the weekend, she suffered painfully the analyst's absence. I was aware of the resistive aspects of the idealization, but I did not interpret them at this time. One day she complained about a Kleinian-oriented lecture that she had attended, which had emphasized the importance in treatment of bringing out the analysand's aggression. She hated what she heard, as it reminded her of caustic confrontations from a previous therapist "accusing" her of hiding anger behind a congenial facade. To be sure, Beverly's idealization of me was, in part, serving to ward off her recognition of destructive impulses toward me. But, more importantly, at that phase in the analysis, as I saw it, she was desperately attempting through idealization to find and to preserve a safe connection to me in the transference. Therefore, I limited my interpretation at that time to asking her if she was frightened that, if she were not continually watchful of herself, this treatment would break down as had two previous ones. She was monitoring herself carefully to protect the analysis from catastrophe. Beverly welcomed this observation and, while it helped relieve her of anxiety to some extent, she still had to restrain any hint of aggression for some time.

Vignette I: (tenth month) acting in

Interpretation of unacknowledged erotic transference

While the patient's behavior and associations had become somewhat less inhibited in the previous few months, I had been noting in recent days that she had returned to being physically reserved with me. For example, she had been closing the outer door to the waiting room very carefully so as not to make a sound. Also, her gait had become sluggish and awkward. Occasionally she caught her hand bag on the door knob, or her heel on the area rug in front of the couch. In a Monday hour, during the tenth month of the analysis, I was given an opportunity to understand and interpret this inhibited, presumably symptomatic behavior.

Beverly had been speaking in the hour of her oldest daughter, a 22-year-old dancer, and of the pleasure that she had gotten over the weekend as she and her husband had watched the daughter perform in a show. About halfway through the hour, Beverly developed a cramp in her leg. Startled by it, she jumped to a half-sitting position and began to rub her leg vigorously, saying with embarrassment:

PATIENT: I got a cramp … Ouch!

ANALYST: [As the cramp subsided and she settled back down on the couch] You looked very much in pain.

P: [Somewhat shyly] That really hurt and besides I hate to be startled.

A: [Notes aloud her embarrassment.]

P: I guess I don't like to be out of control.

A: Out of control?

P: I don't like to move that much here.

A: And yet you seemed to get such pleasure from telling me of your daughter's rhythmic movements.

P: Yes it's wonderful to see her lovely body be so graceful.

[She elaborates more on the pleasure she got and, in contrast, how her own body is awkward.]

A: It seems you can tell me easily and pridefully of your daughter's movements, but you have to be careful not to reveal your own.
P: Yes that's true. I never move much, here.
A: Indeed, to have had such a painful cramp you must have been severely tensing your body, as if to be absolutely sure you did not move, when reminded of your daughter's rhythmic movements.
P: I feel if I move I'm doing something wrong … God this is embarrassing … I feel that I'm not supposed to do this. It feels like I'm doing something wrong.
A: Something wrong?
P: Something sexual … I don't feel guilty exactly … it's just wrong like you wouldn't like it … If you knew what I was doing … the thing is … it's hard to tell you about sexual thoughts … I know in my head that's OK, it's what I'm supposed to do.

[Pause]

A: You are supposed to but you struggle to overcome something in yourself.
P: I'm supposed to tell you what I think.

[Long pause. Very shyly, softly and girlishly]

P: But it's not like a fantasy. That's what I'm afraid of, it really is sexual. I am really doing something sexual. It's like you are doing one thing here and I am doing something else … like that's what I really come for. I know you want me to talk and so I do. I'm always trying to figure out what I can say to get you to talk to me. It's so important that you talk to me. It means so much to me.

This bit of an hour illustrates that, for some time, Beverly had been hiding, while secretly enjoying, erotic feeling and fantasies in response to my presence and voice. This acting-in was now intensifying at this point in the treatment. Symptomatic acts, e.g., bumping her hand bag into the door knob and catching her heel in the area rug, both concealed and reflected conflict between bodily display, aggression and the desire to get caught. Also, these acts drew my attention to her body and its movements, suggesting an unconsciously seductive intent. Beverly's wish to be sexual and displaying is displaced through her allusion to her daughter, with whom unconsciously she is identified.

I understood her narrative of pleasurably watching her daughter dance as a metaphor for her own repressed and inhibited sexuality and exhibitionism. I considered the cramping foot to be a symptomatic act through which she was inviting empathy and interpretation. I contrasted aloud her presentation of herself, lying tensely motionless on the couch with her identificatory pleasure in viewing her daughter's graceful body. Confirmation for the interpretive work appears in the latter part of the hour where she acknowledges her erotic experience with me, and her embarrassment. "It's hard to tell you sexual thoughts," she said.

In the hours that followed there appears to be further confirmation that interpretation of the transference had widened the analytic window into her erotic life, in particular into her masturbatory fantasies and anxieties. Beverly had managed to bear considerable embarrassment as she continued to tell me, with difficulty, more of her erotic "misbehavior" in the hours. I sensed in her voice and manner that she was dutifully confessing to me. I brought this to her attention. As I became aware that she was projecting onto me a punitive internal object, I eventually pointed out the dual (split) image of me that she held in her mind: I was seen and heard as erotically stimulating on the one hand, but as cruelly disapproving on the other. Then, I pointed out to her that her erotic experience, while pleasurable to her, was nonetheless inhibited in that, consciously, she desired no physical contact. She was content; in fact she preferred to be secretly "sexual" in front of me: In other words, she was privately savoring a masturbatory fantasy in which she controlled a maternal presence that simultaneously soothed and excited her, but that easily could be lost. She guiltily revealed that she had taken my voice inside of herself, and was thereby inside of me, controlling the mother-analyst from within.

Transference interpretation yielding fragments of recall

This insight seemed to offer her considerable relief, as she pondered why she preferred this form of pleasure to intercourse with her husband. Soon associations came to mind in which she could not distinguish fantasy from memory: She is a little girl sitting on a man's lap. She is not certain who the man is. Maybe it is her father, she surmises. She is feeling good, sexual. They are pretending to be doing something else, but it is sexual. She likes it very much. She continues to be uncertain whether she is recalling or imagining these events. She cannot really believe, nor does she want to believe, that the man is her father. Over the next two months this "fantasy" came up several more times, each time in a slightly modified version. The final one, at that stage in the treatment, entailed her climbing on father's lap and his saying to her, "Oh so you want more of that do you?" This taunt, in which he totally denied his desire for her, caused Beverly to feel utterly humiliated for having assumed, presumptuously, that her father had wanted her. (Silently, I thought that her "being secretly sexual" with me was a re-living of this quasi-dissociated experience with her father, but with the roles reversed. She had been using my voice and presence for erotic stimulation while pretending to be interested in free association.) Eventually a transference paradigm emerged in which she fantasized herself to be a seductive omnipotent child, while construing me to be a potentially withdrawing, controlled, shocked and invaded father. This paradigm alternated with my being the jealous mother or sister from whose vengeful attacks she must protect herself.

Vignette II: (second year) a dream

A cannibalistic fantasy emerging in the transference

By the time the analysis had entered its second year, another important element had been added to the developing picture of Beverly's erotic fantasy life, one which was introduced over time, intermixed with shame and embarrassment: It seems that Beverly was using "violent", "disgusting" fantasies to help arouse herself during intercourse. These included being tortured and dismembered by violent monster-men. Shame and disgust over these fantasies had caused her to avoid intercourse with her husband whenever she could.

Partly through recall, and in part through reconstruction, a picture of Beverly's early life had developed in which it became clear that her mother's mix of emotional and excessive anxiety and physical exhaustion had led Beverly later to avidly pursue her oedipal father, hoping to meet unfilled pre-oedipal maternal needs from him. While it was not yet clear, at this time, whether Beverly had been recalling a repressed memory of sexual contact with her father, which she placed at age four, or whether she had recalled a repressed fantasy, father had emerged from the associations as stubbornly withholding, overstimulating and given to temper tantrums.

In the hour prior to the dream that follows, Beverly told me anxiously that when she felt shaky she would like to have me hold her. This wish represented a significant development in the transference. In previous hours she had spoken of how much she had liked to have her hand held by family members. Eventually, she told me that she imagined my holding her hand. But this was the first time that she had wanted to be held tightly in my arms. Her associations made it clear to me that the consistent analysis of her transference resistances had revealed the development of an intense and conflicted pre-oedipal maternal transference.

A dream and its interpretation seem to have ushered in a new phase in the analysis. In the dream she goes to my house and someone answers the door. She does not know who this is but she has the impression that it is someone from out of town. She is told that I am not home but that she can wait for me. Then the person leaves the room. Beverly wanders into the kitchen and looks around. She sees some magnets on the refrigerator door. They are sort of ornamental. She takes them in her hands and begins to take them apart, as if fascinated by them. But she can't put them back together. She then becomes fearful that I will come home, see what she has done, and that she will be embarrassed and frightened of my anger.

She then went on to tell me that often when she had left my office she needed to use the ladies room. But usually she refrained because she did not want to reenter the waiting room to obtain the key to the toilet.

A: You don't want to go into the waiting room.

P: No. I am often crying or ruffled and I don't want to be seen that way. Also I don't want to see your next patient. I want to be the only person you see. I know that you have other patients, but I like to pretend that I am the only one. I ignore that you have a personal life.

Mrs. X [a social worker whom she knows] says you are a wonderful teacher, you say things very clearly. It pleases me to hear that she likes you, but I am a little jealous ... I am afraid to tell you these things because it is so intrusive. It makes me feel I don't know how much you can take, what your limits are.

A: As you had felt in the dream?

P: I liked visiting your house, looking around.

A: In the dream, it seems that you were not ignoring that I have a personal life. In fact, you were quite curious about it. Were you freer to move around there and explore your curiosity a bit more than here?

P: Yeah. I liked that but then I got so scared.

A: Scared?

P: Yes, like I had gone too far. I wasn't supposed to touch the magnets.

A: They were off limits?

P: I feel sort of awed by their attraction and how they pull together tightly... It is so fascinating.

A: Friday you let me know how much you wanted me to hold you, how tightly ... Perhaps tightly as magnets.

P: Yes [nodding], very, very tight ... Then I got afraid.

A: Afraid?

P: Yes, what would it be like for you if I gripped you so tightly? Would you pull back and reject me?

A: As if you are afraid that by tight holding you would be invading me and I would pull back to save myself.

P: Yes.

[Nodding with much affect ... She seems to wait expectantly for me to say more.]

A: Through the dream you seem to be finding the room to explore just how safe it might be for you and I to fit together as tightly as magnets. If both of us are drawn equally to the other, you can be sure that I would not push you away in fear that you were invading me.

[P continues to nod enthusiastically as I talk. Much body movement is observable for the first time.]

A: How does it work? How can tight, close contact be safe?

[P moves and smiles.]

P: I want you to know how good it is when you can understand me this way and say things I can't find words for. So often I can't even find the words to know myself what I feel.

At the beginning of the hour Beverly had said that she was quite anxious. I did not encourage her to associate to more of the dream elements, although the theme of rivalry for me with other women was obvious. Additionally, I privately associated the magnets with sexuality, male genitals, the desire to separate mother from father and merger wishes toward mother. Because her anxiety over her fantasy to invade my body was so intense, I felt it needed immediate attention. It is noteworthy that although invasiveness anxieties regarding erotic oedipal wishes toward father had emerged earlier in the analysis, these current longings seemed to have to do with entering the mother's body; they appeared more regressive and primitive.

A veritable flood of material confirming the interpretive work followed over the next several weeks. For example, the next day Beverly dreamed of happily cleaning messes, apparently a reaction formation for her aggressive and rivalrous wishes expressed in the Monday hour. Associations concerning her being overly accommodating to her physical therapy clients' requests emerged, reflecting regressive merger wishes toward them to ward off anxiety about rivalry, aggression and separation.

I offered Beverly the interpretation that she apparently had wanted to create with her clients an illusion of oneness, as if to encourage them to feel that they were inside of her, as she had wanted to be inside of me. But then she would become terrified that at any moment I would ragefully expel her to save my life. She confirmed this with many associations over the next several weeks.

By my continuing to interpret her transference wishes to be held and their attendant anxieties we learned that she wanted to be held while she sat on the floor because she needed a solid foundation that would contain her feeling of "falling apart". She especially wanted to be held at the end of an hour to be reassured that she had not destroyed me. If she could take a sensory impression of me with her, she could hope to counteract her fear that a vitally needed mother-analyst would be lost and that, subsequently, she would be "lost in space."

Controlling a monster: emergence of the father transference

Many associations indicated that previously warded off cannibalistic fantasies were emerging in the transference. For example, after saying that thoughts are "too hot to touch" Beverly thought of a science fiction movie in which an alien life form invades and agitates people, like a spinning cyclone inside of them. When I suggested that perhaps she experienced herself as a cyclone inside of me, she immediately recalled that she had destroyed what she wanted most when she told sister and mother about sexual activities with father. After that everybody hated her. She wanted to be held to keep from shaking apart by a flood of terrifying memories.

Now another aspect of the defensive purpose of the idealization of the analyst had become clear: She was afraid that monster-men, werewolves (oral sadistic cannibals), would get her and take advantage of her for their own purpose. "I am afraid that I will turn you into my dad," she said. She feels loathsome, cruel. "I tried to torture my mother for not taking care of me. I want to hold you at the end of the hour to know that I haven't destroyed you with my rage." In an hour two days later, the material deepens still further:

P: I can see you in different roles, either as the aggressor or you just don't care—as the enemy. So I try to get out of that state before the hour ends.

A: Perhaps when you want me to hold you, you are trying to reassure yourself that I am not an enemy.

P: I have an image that I hold onto that is really crucial. In this other frame of mind you are the aggressor (Father) or you are preoccupied (Mother). I get very angry like this—massive rage. Like you become my mother, this person who is too busy to spend time with me. Then what I do is destroy you in my mind. You are wiped out and then I suffer much.

[She cries.]

A: Then you have no one.

P: I wanted you to hold me at the end because I wanted to have something that wouldn't be destroyed.

A: So when you saw me as the enemy you destroyed me. But then, before you left, you wanted physical holding, as if to reassure yourself that you had destroyed me only in your mind, and only temporarily.

P: Yes, exactly. I carry an image of you, the way you look, and your voice—a nice image. When I destroy you, you are a figure on the blackboard and I erase you. Like the image of my father. You became the one who doesn't take care of me, who doesn't protect me.

I got so enraged at my mother at a young age. I tried to get even, to torture her for not taking care of me.

[She cries.]

P: It's like a kid carrying a teddy bear. If a parent does or doesn't do something they destroy it in a rage and there is nothing. Then I think, "What have I done?"

Discussion

Clinical implications

One technical advantage of bringing to center stage fantasy that predates the trauma is that doing so facilitates recall. The fantasy which the child imported to her incestuous experience may first be made conscious and partially worked through in a transference context, such as the maternal transference, which is significantly less terrifying than the raw recall of the trauma proper—i.e., at a moment when the child had been utterly unsupported. The following sequence of analytic work facilitating recall is a frequent occurrence:

1 The analysand projects or acts in a frightening unconscious fantasy, often of pre-oedipal origin, into the transference while warding off its recognition (resistance).
2 The analyst perceives the fantasy encoded in the associations and experiences it through introjective identification.
3 The analyst interprets the transference.
4 The analysand, through insight and initial working through, survives the sequence (experiences safety).
5 When the work in the transference somewhat detoxifies the fantasy, the associations to it facilitate recall of the abuse.

Beverly is representative of those patients who initially bring hysterical-looking symptomatology and psychodynamics to the analysis. Further into the work, however, a more complex picture manifests itself in which pre-oedipal difficulties play themselves out on the oedipal field. In the example presented here, Beverly's ill and tired mother could not be available sufficiently to assist her in the first months and years of life to develop, adequately, a cohesive self. Beverly, therefore, used pervasive masturbatory fantasies to help maintain her sense of aliveness and her tie to her mother. The content of these fantasies involved entering mother's body while she slept and devouring her (cannibalizing her). Later, as an oedipal-age child, she rushed to her sexually seductive father, overtly to be recognized by him, to be picked up. Unconsciously, she was displacing her need for pre-oedipal maternal care to him.

Reconstruction suggests that the collusive enactment began with the oedipal father responding to his maternally deprived daughter's eager presentation of herself to him, with bodily closeness and stroking of her non-genital body parts. As the caressing began gently, it was pleasurable and non-threatening to the girl. In fact, the child had felt, initially, that she was finally receiving the caring ministrations that were all too infrequently delivered by her mother. As the sensations, presumably for each participant, became increasingly erotic, each pretended not to notice what they were doing together, perhaps even feigning to be interested in a television show that they were watching. It is as if this collusion had initiated a jointly shared dissociated state in which the left hand, as it were, pretended not to notice what the right hand was doing. When the father touched the child's genitals, her arousal guiltily heightened. But she remained, still, a willing participant. (See Gullestad, 2005 for a discussion of gentle parental seductions and the child as a willing accomplice.) Eventually, something happened that she could not have been prepared for: She sensed father losing control of himself in his arousal, as his fingers or penis began to push against her genitals. While it remains uncertain in her mind whether her father had actually penetrated her, she now became terrified of a dreadful intrusion as she began to feel used and out of control, both of the situation and of her bodily spaces. Her longing for intimate tenderness had been met by a dreadful mismatch of her father's behavior (see Ferenczi, 1933). Instead of finding mildly erotic excitement in a context of warm, sensual, displaced maternal interaction that unconsciously she had longed for, she had been subjected to a horrifying transformation: It was as if father, in his heightening arousal, had burst out of his skin to become a non-human, i.e., a ravenous, invading monster, later to be symbolized as a creature from outer space. Her father and mother's frequently observed fights, her unresolved rage toward her mother and her terrifying erotic collusions with her father combined to re-stimulate masturbatory fantasies that had taken on an increasingly sadomasochistic cast.

The erotic enactment with her father, then, signaled the return of an envious, vengeful, retaliatory, internal mother. It therefore had to be subdued through inhibition and dissociation. Her sexuality was thereby impaired throughout adolescence and married life. The inhibition had been shaped, as well, by identifications with part objects of both genders: In this fantasy she was a ravenously hungry, devouring mouth-vagina-infant and a boring clitoris-penis-father. This composite manifested itself in the wish and terror of penetrating the body of the analyst-mother and stealing his life-supporting supplies. Finally, another version of the frightening and guilt-provoking cannibalistic fantasy emerged in which she, herself, was a monster, a werewolf, who had invaded the mother's body (in the analysis, the mother-father-analyst) to steal life-giving supplies, an act which would easily result in mother's death since she was sickly, tired and enfeebled.

Comments on erotic transference

While Freud (1920) viewed erotized transference love through a variety of lenses, first and foremost he saw it as resistance. Even more, he and subsequent writers such as Betty Joseph (1993) have described patients' erotic love exclusively as a destructive vehicle for attacking the analyst's efforts to conduct an analysis. The case illustration in this chapter indeed substantiates the warnings of these writers to attend assiduously to the destructive intent behind the erotization and idealization of the analyst. But I argue here for the vital necessity to recognize and to appreciate another aspect of the patient's unconscious agenda. The woman via erotic and idealized transference love is making a valorous and successful effort to survive psychically, by maintaining hope, by escaping depression and by evading terror. In the search for the idealized father-analyst the woman is enacting her struggle with an inner maternal presence that simultaneously must be sought and escaped. She is sought to consolidate the self, that is, to enhance life, while paradoxically she is fled from to avoid death—that is, to prevent an immersion in what to the child seems like mother's immanent psychic collapse. Father, then, represents a savior from a merger with a dead mother (Green, 1983).

Summary

For Freud, the traumatic factor was always an admixture of an event(s) external to the ego, originating from the environment or the drive, and the mind's construal of what the event meant to the subject. His insistence that trauma has meaning, and that it is the meaning that is the traumatic factor, has remained a mainstay of the psychoanalytic position, regardless of theoretical orientation. This position distinguishes *psychoanalytic* trauma theory from earlier views and from those stemming from contemporary neuroscience. (See Diamond in this volume for a fuller description of this distinction.) In this contribution I have argued that a child's mind, while being abused, does not respond as a passive tabula rasa simply recording or dissociating what is happening to her. Rather, the child imports to abusive encounters with adults drive-related fantasies from earlier in life. In the case that I have presented here these fantasies had provoked intense unconscious guilt co-determining, with other factors, what she was experiencing. As well, they contributed to a guilty character development. Recognizing and interpreting these fantasies as they emerge in psychoanalytic transferences can greatly further the treatment and may, uniquely, provide the necessary leverage for the difficult task of recognizing and working through primitive forms of guilt.

Notes

1 A briefer version of this chapter won the Jean B. Sanville award for creative writing in psychoanalysis given by the Los Angeles Institute and Society for Psychoanalytic Studies (LAISPS). It was also presented at the 44th International Psychoanalytical Association Congress in Rio de Janeiro, Brazil, 2005.

2 Additional comments on my interpretive stance with this patient can be found elsewhere (see Spivak, 2014). A detailed account of my views on the interpretive process is also available elsewhere (see Spivak, 2011).

References

Bohleber, W. (2010). *Destructiveness, Intersubjectivity, and Trauma: The Identity Crisis of Modern Psychoanalysis.* London: Karnac.

Botella, C. & Botella, S. (2005). *The Work of Psychic Figurability: Mental States without Representation.* Hove & New York: Brunner-Routledge.

Bromberg, P.M. (1998). *Standing In the Spaces: Essays on Clinical Process, Trauma, and Dissociation.* Hillsdale, NJ: Analytic Press.

Balint, M. (1969). Trauma and object relationship. *International Journal of Psychoanalysis,* 50: 429–435.

Bigras, J. (1990). Psychoanalysis as incestuous repetition: Some technical considerations. *Adult Analysis and Childhood Sexual Abuse,* H.B. Levine (ed.), Hillsdale, NJ: Analytic Press, 73–196.

Blum, H.P. (1987). The role of identification in the resolution of trauma. *Psychoanalytic Quarterly,* 56: 609–627.

Bollas, C. (1987). *The Shadow of the Object.* London: Free Association Books.

Civitarese, G. (2013). *The Violence of Emotions: Bion and Post-Bionian Psychoanalysis.* London: Routledge.

Davies, J.M. & Frawley, M.G. (1994). *Treating the Adult Survivor of Childhood: A Sexual Abuse Psychoanalytic Perspective.* New York: Basic Books.

Fairbairn, W.R.D. (1943). The repression and the return of bad objects (with special reference to the "war neuroses"). *Psychoanalytic Studies of the Personality.* London: Karnac, 1952, 59–81.

Fenichel, O. (1937). The concept of trauma in contemporary psychoanalytic theory. *The collected papers of Otto Fenichel,* H. Fenichel & D. Rapaport (eds.) (2nd Series). New York: Norton, 1954, 49–69.

Ferenczi, S. (1933). Confusion of tongues between adults and the child. *Final Contributions to the Problems and Methods of Psychoanalysis.* New York: Basic Books, 1955, 156–167.

Freud, S. (1900). The interpretation of dreams. *Standard Edition 20.* London: Hogarth Press.

Freud, S. (1920). Beyond the pleasure principle. *Standard Edition 18.* London: Hogarth Press.

Freud, S. (1936). *The Problem of Anxiety.* New York: Psychoanalytic Quarterly Press & Norton.

Green, A. (1983). The dead mother. *On Private Madness.* Madison, CT: International Universities Press, 1986.

Gullestad, S.E. (2005). Who is "who" in dissociation? A plea for psychodynamics in a time of trauma. *International Journal of Psychoanalysis,* 86: 639–656.

Joseph, B. (1993). On transference some current observations. *On Freud's "Observations on Transference-Love",* S. Person *et al.* (eds.). New Haven: Yale University Press.

Kernberg, O. (1976). *Object Relations Theory and Clinical Psychoanalysis.* New York: Jason Aronson.

Klein, M. (1975). *Envy and Gratitude.* London: Hogarth Press & Institute of Psychoanalysis.

Levine, H.B. (2012). The colourless canvas: Representation, therapeutic action and the creation of mind. *International Journal of Psychoanalysis*, 93: 607–629.

Schafer, R. (1992). *Retelling a Life.* New York: Basic Books.

Spivak, A.P. (2011). The interpretive act: Returning freedom and agency to a beleaguered ego. *The Second Century of Psychoanalysis: Evolving Perspective on Therapeutic Action*, M.J. Diamond & C. Christian (eds.). London: Karnac.

Spivak, A.P. (2014). The interpretive process: The power of "mere" words. *Journal of the American Psychoanalytic Association*, 62(6): 1063–1073.

Stern, D.B. (2003). *Unformulated Experience: From Dissociation to Imagination in Psychoanalysis.* Hillsdale, NJ: Analytic Press.

Index